banishing
the
blues

banishing
the
blues

Hilary Boyd

Medical consultant Dr Hagen Rampes BSc MBChB MRCPsych

Inspirational ways to improve your mood

MITCHELL BEAZLEY

Banishing the Blues
Hilary Boyd

Published in 2000 by Mitchell Beazley,
an imprint of Octopus Publishing Group Ltd
2–4 Heron Quays, London, E14 4JP

Publisher's note
This book is intended only for people suffering from low
mood states and not for those suffering from medically
diagnosed depression. Before following any advice or
exercises contained in this book, it is recommended that
you consult your doctor if you suffer from any health
problems or special conditions. The publishers cannot
accept responsibility for any injuries or damage incurred
as a result of following the advice given in this book.

ISBN 1 84000 315 4

A CIP catalogue copy of this book is available from the
British Library.

Commissioning Editor	Vivien Antwi
Executive Art Editor	Kenny Grant
Project Editor	Chloë Garrow
Editor	Claire Musters
Designer	Miranda Harvey
Illustration	Trina Dalziel, Miranda Harvey
Picture research	Helen Stallion
Proofreader	Laura Harper
Indexer	Diana le Core
Production	Catherine Lay

Printed and bound by Toppan Printing Company, China
Typeset in Frutiger & Foundry

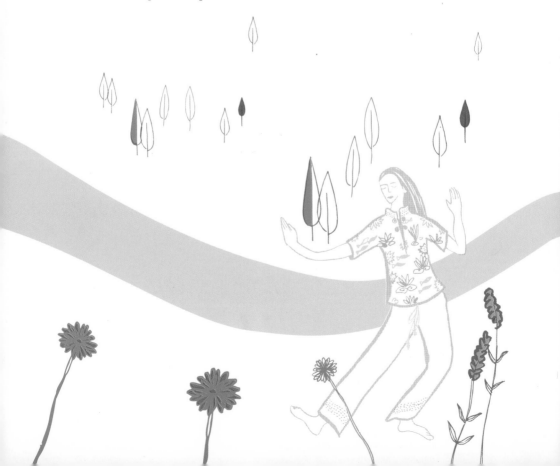

Contents

Introduction

We all feel blue sometimes – it is part of life. But please don't despair. There are so many ways we can help ourselves when we feel down, especially when we understand the mechanism of our low mood and are aware of all our treatment options.

Depression affects a third of the population at some time in their lives. But many of us would far rather admit to heart disease or cancer than to being depressed. We see it as a social stigma, believing mental dysfunction, even of a temporary nature, as akin to madness. We are too ashamed to admit it. We even feel it might be our fault. If we suspect we might be depressed we either just miserably sit it out, or take medication such as Prozac and wait for it to go away. But with so many of us suffering from depression today, it is time to radically alter this way of thinking. Rather than blaming ourselves, or just taking medication and expecting it to go away, we must look at the wider picture to see why we might be susceptible to an attack in the first place.

Although there is more research looking into depression nowadays than there has ever been, the definitive cause, a reliable diagnostic system, and the best way to treat the disease still elude researchers and the medical profession. One of the reasons for this is that the disease has so many different symptoms, from panic attacks and sleeplessness to appetite loss and the psychological problems of low self-esteem. Some of the symptoms that may be present in one person are not found in

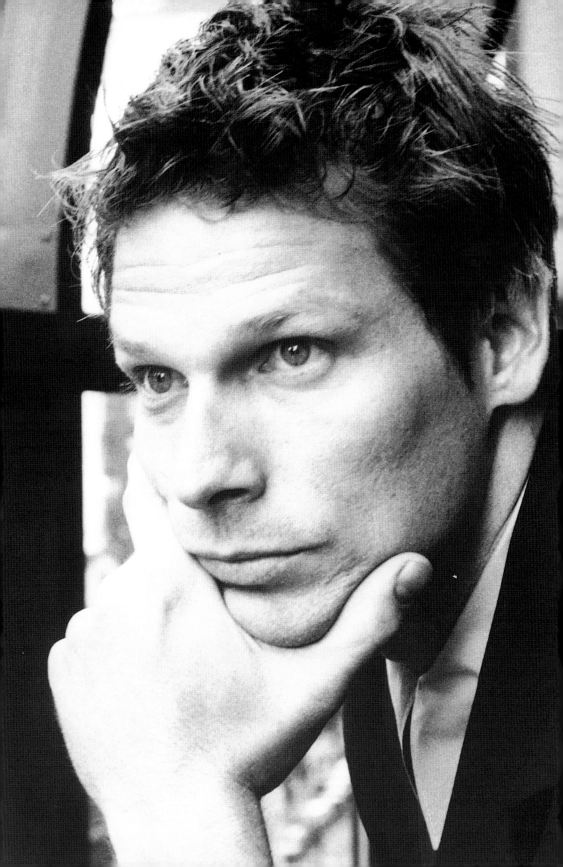

others and some suffer from many symptoms, while others only show a few. There are degrees of depression: mild, moderate, and severe, with bipolar, or manic depression, being placed in a separate category altogether. There are also trigger factors that are associated with the disease – biology, psychology, and the environment – which are thought to combine in some way to produce the condition, but research is still not clear as to why or how depression should occur in one person and not in another when the same factors are present in both their lives.

So what should we do if we feel low and our mood persists for no reason that we can understand? Do we have to reach for the Prozac without delay? Obviously if your depression is so severe that you are totally incapacitated by it, or if you are suffering from bipolar disorder, then antidepressant drugs can be a suitable, and, in many cases, successful, treatment. But if your depression is mild or moderate then there are many things, including nutrition, exercise, therapies, and techniques such as visualization and meditation, that can work to alleviate your depression. And not only can these therapies help to treat an existing condition, but they can also make a recurrence of depression less likely in the future.

This book is divided into two sections. The first, "Knowing your own mind", explains what happens to our brains and our bodies when we are depressed and outlines the possible causes of depression. The main part of the book "Ways to improve your mood" begins by discussing the importance of nutrition as this can be a major contributory factor – some experts believe that up to 70 per cent of depression is food-related, caused by sensitivities to food such as wheat, sugar, and dairy products.

The section then goes on to offer information and advice about alternative treatments which boost the immune system, shed light on our mental and spiritual processes, reduce unhelpful stress, and make us as strong as possible in mind, body, and spirit to minimize the devastating effects of depression in our lives both now and in the future. Such things as yoga, colour therapy, and journalling are covered. The basic details of how these therapies work are given, so that anyone who is interested in them, whether they suffer from depression or not, can benefit from reading this book. For example, if you have a very stressful job try the stress-reducing techniques on pages 98–101. The text also explains how each of the therapies can specifically help to alleviate the symptoms of depression and an at-a-glance colour-coding system on each of these pages instantly tells you which symptoms the particular treatment can help with (see key, right).

It is so important to understand that there is no reason to feel ashamed if we do suffer from low mood states as we are not alone. And there are avenues of help out there that can support us both mentally and physically. Once we realize this, depression need not be such a frightening experience. And those around us who do not suffer any of the symptoms themselves will be able to be much more informed and sympathetic too.

Hilary Bayd

Key to tabs

Sadness

Anxiety

Fatigue

Irritability

Insomnia

Low self-esteem

Apathy

The bars above are used throughout the "Ways to improve your mood" section to indicate what symptoms in particular the therapy can relieve.

Knowing your own mind

Feelings and meanings

Our moods change constantly, and everything we do is affected by them. Each one of us experiences good moods when we feel happy and things are going well. But we also all have bad moods, when we are angry or are fed up. These mood patterns also have many variations in between, such as boredom, irritation, contentment, and joy. For most of us, our so-called "normal" mood is a day-to-day balance of these emotions. But sometimes that balance becomes upset and tips into a prolonged low mood that, if accompanied by certain symptoms, is medically categorized as depression.

The problem with depression is that it is difficult to define. Unlike other illnesses, it has no clear diagnostic test. This presents two major problems: a person suffering from depression may not be aware that she or he needs help, and the doctor, when faced with a depressed patient, may fail to diagnose the real problem. However, psychiatrists have now settled on a number of symptoms for depression. Not everyone who is depressed will show all the symptoms, and the degree to which they are affected will vary.

Depression can be a bewildering state. We often think that we are "feeling low" and should just snap out of it. There is also a stigma attached to any form of mental illness, which may make us ashamed to talk about the way we feel. It is important to explore the symptoms so that we can recognize the difference between just feeling "blue" and depression. With this knowledge we can identify how we feel, which will help us to seek support and treatment when we need it.

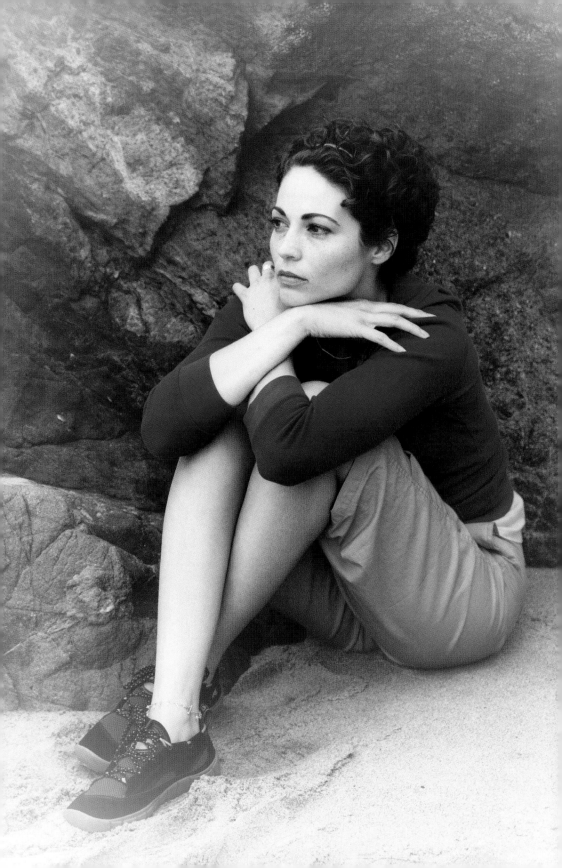

How do moods vary?

If you have ever suffered from depression, then the difference between just a passing unhappiness and real depression will be painfully obvious to you. But for those who are not familiar with the problem it can be more difficult to pick up on the symptoms, so here we explore how you can differentiate between being merely in a passing low mood and being depressed.

Gender differences

Studies done in Great Britain in 1995 show that women get depressed almost twice as much as men do. No one knows for certain why this is so. And mixed anxiety and depression occurs in 9.9% of females, while it only affects 5.4% of males. However, men are three times more likely than women to become dependent on drugs and alcohol.

What does a temporary low mood feel like?

If we are suffering from passing low moods then we may feel tired and irritable. We may also find it difficult to do some of the routine things like going to work, washing up, or making a phone call to a relative. We might also snap at family or work colleagues. We have all experienced times of feeling like this and, while they might last a day or two, a chat to a good friend or a diverting event will quickly bring us back to our usual selves.

There are, of course, life events that naturally trigger negative moods. The sadness we feel when something unpleasant happens, such as a family death or losing our job, is normal and is actually an important part of the grieving process. If we don't express anger and sadness at these events then our bottled up emotions may come back to haunt us, sometimes years later.

We all worry about things to a certain extent. These may be serious things, such as the mortgage, or less serious, such as a daughter's performance in a school play. But the anxiety does pass. Depression, however, is often accompanied by high levels of anxiety that do not seem to have a specific cause. Everything makes us anxious, sometimes to the degree that we cannot go out or face other people.

Major characteristics of depression

Depression, whether categorized as mild, moderate, or severe, does have a few distinctive features. Loss of self-esteem can indicate depression and sufferers often feel worthless, thinking that everything bad that is happening to them is their own fault, and that somehow they deserve what they are going through.

When we are unhappy, we usually know the cause of it and our negative thoughts are focused on the unwanted life event. But when we are depressed our negative thoughts are not necessarily based in reality. And these negative thoughts will trigger more negative thought, however unrealistic, in an ever-downward spiral. Mere unhappiness passes; quite soon we feel different, even if a little sadness lingers. But depression seems to go on forever, and every day seems like an eternity. It is also extremely difficult to be comforted while we are in depression. If we are desperately unhappy about something, there is nothing we want more than to be hugged and held as we cry and talk about how we feel. It doesn't make our sadness disappear, but it does help. This comfort is not available to a depressed person, because depression makes all forms of love and compassion inaccessible. We can hear the person asking what's wrong, can see the person's concern written on their face, can even feel their arms around us, but we are completely isolated inside our depression.

Normal unhappiness is a state of mind but depression is an illness. It has acknowledged symptoms and treatments, even if doctors cannot confirm the diagnosis by taking a blood sample. But even those of us who do realize we are depressed may not seek help, because we feel we should be able to make ourselves better. But we wouldn't think that if we had pneumonia would we?

Depression in other people

Another important reason for learning the distinction between unhappiness and depression is so that we can recognize it in others. Living with a depressed person can be extremely difficult. No amount of "Pull yourself together", or "What have you got to be depressed about?" will have the slightest effect – indeed, if these phrases are repeated too often frustration and irritation can set in, isolating the ill person even further in their misery.

It is not always easy to persuade someone who is depressed to seek help. But understanding the problem and the possible treatments will reduce the frustration and can eventually result in the sufferer getting the help they need. What is clear is that there are now many accessible strategies for alleviating the symptoms of depression once the condition has been recognized.

How depression can affect your feelings
"I thought that the way I felt would pass, that I'd wake up one morning and be my old self, but nothing made me laugh any more, not even my own children. I began to feel that they would be better off without me. Nobody could understand what I had to be miserable about. There wasn't a reason for it, but I was still shut in a horrible blackness and my life seemed to have no point."

What is depression?

Depression is becoming alarmingly common – it has even been labelled the "common cold" of psychiatric problems. Epidemiological studies suggest that between 15 and 30 per cent of the world's population will experience a bout of depression at some time in their lives. Imagine the toll this takes on relationships, work, and an overstretched medical service. So what exactly is it?

The main symptoms of depression

- Anxiety attacks
- Change in eating habits
- Difficulty in concentrating and making decisions
- Disturbed sleep patterns
- Feelings of despair and hopelessness
- Irritability and impatience with others
- Lack of energy and being tired constantly
- Lack of enjoyment in things that previously gave pleasure
- Loss of self-esteem and general confidence
- Loss of sex drive
- Ongoing low mood
- Persistent negative thoughts
- Self-criticism
- Self-destructive behaviour
- Thoughts of suicide

A definition of depression

"Depression" is a medical term that is used to describe a wide range of mood disorders that create psychological distress in the sufferer. But because of the variety and degree of symptoms, and the fact that everyone is affected in different ways, depression has been difficult to define. It was not until the start of the 20th century that doctors began to work on classifications and a diagnosis. Until recently, psychiatrists classified a person's depression as either "endogenous" or "exogenous".

Endogenous depression, taken from the Greek word meaning "growing within", describes the illness when there is no apparent cause. It is assumed then that the depression has a purely biological origin. This type of depression is often referred to as "clinical" depression, and is seen as the most severe. Exogenous depression, commonly known as "reactive" depression, describes, on the other hand, depression that is caused by some traumatic event such as bereavement, divorce, or losing a job.

Nowadays, the experts agree that these classifications are actually inadequate, as many people's symptoms blur the line between the two. They prefer to divide depression into three categories: mild, moderate, or severe, using widely accepted diagnostic systems that go by the number and degree of symptoms present in a patient at any one time. These systems are seen as a general guideline only, as people still rarely fall neatly into one of these categories. And even with these guidelines, many doctors fail to diagnose depression in their patients because they treat the specific symptoms, such as sleeping difficulties, without looking at the broader picture.

Possible causes

Alongside the general classification of mild, moderate, and severe, there are further categories, based on circumstances, that could cause the illness. The three most common contexts are childbirth, seasonal light deprivation, and manic depression.

Postnatal Depression is experienced by some women in the weeks following childbirth. This is thought to be brought on by the sudden drop in hormone levels in the mother's body after the birth, but there is still no real understanding as to why some women are affected while others are not. And it is a mystery that some of the women who suffer from it are affected after one pregnancy, but not after another. Psychological and social factors may play a part, but there is no research yet to prove this.

Seasonal Affective Disorder (SAD) is a recognized disorder in which the person affected suffers regular depressive bouts every year when the daylight diminishes during winter months (see pages 116–17).

Manic Depression is also known as bipolar (relating to two extremes) affective disorder, because the sufferer experiences not only depression but also mania – over-excitement, hyperactivity, and delusional thoughts – in unpredictable cycles.

Symptoms of depression

It is generally agreed that depression consists of a persistent low mood, which is accompanied by at least five of the symptoms listed in the box on the left, and has lasted for two weeks or more. For some people it comes on suddenly, while for others it creeps up gradually without the sufferers being fully aware of it.

The number and severity of symptoms varies from person to person. A sufferer may also display physical symptoms such as nausea, difficulty in breathing, headaches, stomach cramps, and dizziness. And, unfortunately, these physical manifestations can throw a doctor off the scent if he or she does not make a psychological evaluation as well. There are also physical illnesses that can present themselves as depression because they have similar symptoms, such as anaemia, hypothyroidism, and cancer.

The DALY scale

Disability-adjusted life year, or DALY, is a scale that is used to measure global disease, and it combines the levels of disability and premature death. Respiratory and gut infections have consistently been at the top of this list to date, but a study from Harvard University and WHO Global Burden of Disease predicts that depression will be number two on the list by the year 2020.

Symptoms explored

It is important to understand what depressive symptoms might feel like to the sufferer. Most of the emotions listed below are experienced by all of us at one time or another, but, whether they are due to stress or a traumatic event, those moments do eventually pass and we get back to feeling normal. Only occasionally do the symptoms accumulate, making us fall victim to depression.

Helping ourselves

Whether someone is mildly, moderately, or severely depressed they will need a sensitive assessment carried out by a professional and then the appropriate action can be taken. However, we can also do a lot ourselves to alleviate the symptoms of mild or moderate depression, as well as help to prevent it in the future.

Depression is not just a sleepless night or a row with your partner. As stated before, it is an accumulation of at least five of the symptoms listed here, which appear over a period longer than two weeks. And depression can either start suddenly, within a few days or weeks, or take months to develop. So what are the possible warning signs?

Anxiety attacks Many people suffer from anxiety attacks without being depressed. But it is common for depression to be accompanied by high levels of anxiety. For instance, you might be convinced that your neighbourhood has suddenly become intensely dangerous and become too frightened to go out as a result. You may, alternatively, find yourself sitting on a train and suddenly your heart starts racing, you become sweaty and short of breath, and feel extremely vulnerable in your environment, although there is no obvious reason why you should.

Change in eating habits You may go off your food and lose weight. Nothing looks tempting; you are hungry, but when you see the food on your plate you lose your appetite and feel nauseous. Alternatively, you may eat too much and put on weight. Food becomes a comfort and you turn to it to fill your emotional emptiness. This works for a few minutes, but then you are disgusted with yourself and your low mood returns. You may take on compulsive eating patterns, like bingeing or purging.

Difficulty in concentrating and making decisions We all have moments in which we can't concentrate but they may be happening more often than usual to you. For example, you read the paper and realize you can't remember a thing that is on the page you've just read. Your work seems to take you twice as long as it used to. Normal indecisiveness and forgetfulness can be a direct result of having too much to do, which means you can't concentrate on anything properly, but this is more ongoing.

Disturbed sleep patterns You may have trouble getting to sleep. You may wake very early and not be able to get back to sleep. The latter is very common in depression and can be particularly upsetting because everyone else is asleep and you feel isolated and exhausted, knowing you have a busy day, but are too tired to face it. No amount of staying up late to make yourself extra tired before going to bed helps the situation.

Feelings of despair and hopelessness These feelings can be frightening and overwhelming. Happy memories turn sour. The present feels dead and neverending and the future seems to

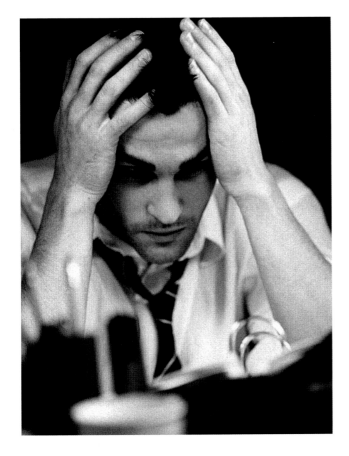

Depression is often bewildering for the sufferer because there are so many different and unfamiliar feelings involved that they may become agitated and confused.

Mild depression

This may be indicated by five or six symptoms. The person affected will still be working and functioning at home, but with reduced usefulness and taking no pleasure in what he or she is doing.

Moderate depression

This may be indicated by six or more symptoms of increased severity. The sufferer will probably not be working, or will be experiencing trouble at work, and will also have become isolated from their social life and family activities.

hold nothing for you but bleakness. There just doesn't seem to be any point to your life. You want to give up and run away, to avoid facing the next day. You can be sitting watching a programme on television and all of a sudden just burst into tears and feel a flood of misery wash over you. The worst thing is, you can't explain why you feel this way.

Irritability and impatience with others You feel like shouting at everyone, and don't seem able to stop yourself from doing so. You might find those close to you are frustrated with your negativity but even their words of encouragement drive you mad.

Lack of energy and being tired constantly If your sleep is disturbed then obviously you will feel tired. But this is more than that. It is a fundamental lack of energy to do anything at all except crawl back under the duvet. You can't be bothered to do even the simplest of tasks, such as changing a light bulb.

Lack of enjoyment in things that previously gave pleasure You always used to look forward to taking the children ice-skating on Saturday afternoons. Now you go through the motions but it's just no fun. You try to rationalize your lack of enjoyment by deciding that you are just tired or under stress, but it doesn't really explain the bleakness that surrounds you even when you see your charming five-year-old pirouetting on the ice.

Loss of self-esteem and confidence You feel worthless and your confidence has disappeared. You are sure all your friends and work colleagues, and even the man behind the counter in the delicatessen, are looking down on you and it is difficult to face them. Walking into a room, picking your son up from school, or chairing a meeting – everything is tainted by the feeling that you are just not up to it.

Loss of sex drive Sex is the last thing on your mind. Whatever your previous level of libido, the thought of sex now arouses no interest or desire. Your partner might not be able to see that your problem stems from your depression rather than being a reaction to them. This apparent rejection, unless understood and accommodated, can be the cause of relationship difficulties.

Ongoing low mood We all have bad days, sometimes bad weeks, but your low mood goes on and on, regardless of what sort of a day you've had. You can't remember feeling happy, and you feel perpetually miserable, gloomy, and wretched.

Persistent negative thoughts Friends are thoughtless and don't care. The postman delivers late to spite you. You are too fat, too ugly, and too stupid. You suddenly hate the bedroom curtains, which you adored a few weeks ago. You find yourself putting too negative an emphasis on everything around you.

Self-criticism Somehow you believe that if you were a "better" person, then you wouldn't feel like this. You are convinced that your friend, your partner, and your sister are not plagued by these feelings, because they are successful people, unlike you. You might even think you deserve to feel the way you do.

Self-destructive behaviour Your alcohol intake goes up and you feel you have to have alcohol to survive the day. Maybe you start drinking earlier in the day, or drink all day long. You may take up smoking, or smoke more than you used to. You begin to use illicit drugs in a desperate bid to find oblivion from your misery. The respite is, inevitably, only temporary, and your return to reality is even harder than it was before.

Thoughts of suicide You think about suicide a lot and contemplate the methods you might use to kill yourself. Part of you is sure that no one will care anyway, although the other part knows this isn't true. In extreme cases you can really convince yourself that you will be doing the world a huge favour by dying.

The different levels of depression

As previously stated, there are three categories of depression (see the boxes on the left and right for their definitions). These are only guidelines, as many depressed people overlap two of the categories, or progress from one to another. The terrible loneliness in depression is only exacerbated by the lack of understanding of the condition. If you can realize that your symptoms are part of a recognized disease, just as a headache is a symptom of sinusitis, then you can seek help in a similar way.

Severe depression
This will mean that the sufferer is unable to function at a normal level any more. The most extreme cases might suffer hallucinations and delusions and be at serious risk of committing suicide.

Brain matter

To understand depression we have to look beyond the traumatic life events and environmental influences to examine the contributions that biology and brain function make to the illness as well.

Is there biological evidence of depression in the brain? And is there a specific "depression" hormone or gene? Although the prevailing thought is that depression is a combination of factors, research shows that there are biochemical changes in the brains of many depressed people, such as abnormally low levels of the brain chemicals (called neurotransmitters), and, in some cases, increased levels of the hormone cortisol (see pages 26–7). Modern brain-imaging also highlights changed patterns of activity in the depressed brain. And there is research that implies a genetic predisposition.

The main problem in defining the biology of depression is summed up by that old adage, "which comes first, the chicken or the egg ?". Although there is clear evidence that hormone and brain chemical levels are disrupted in depressed people, to date there is no conclusive research as to whether the changing levels bring about depression, or whether the depression itself acts to alter the levels. And different depressive conditions probably have different biological and brain abnormalities at their root.

Many of these questions are still unanswered, but to understand the current research and the treatments available it helps to have a basic knowledge of the workings of the brain and the systems, chemicals, and hormones that are involved in depressive illnesses.

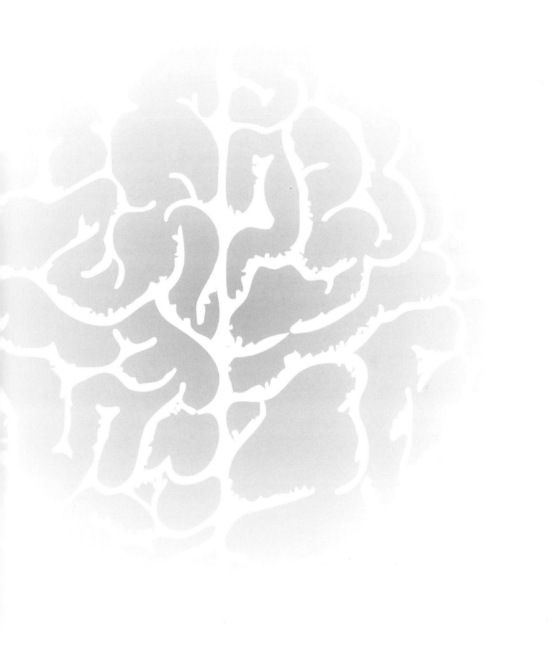

How the brain works

Although familiarity with the complex workings of the brain is not going to explain everything that happens during a depressive episode, it does help us to have some knowledge of the mechanisms that directly affect our brain activity, hormones, and overall mood patterns. So here comes the science. Don't panic if you find it complicated – it is.

The structure of the brain

The brain is basically the body's control centre and it is roughly the size of a melon, although slightly squashed in shape. It is divided into two halves, or hemispheres, and both of these have four parts, also known as lobes. Each of these lobes is associated with a specific function. The frontal lobe is concerned with higher mental processes such as thinking, conceptualizing, and planning while the parietal lobe controls movement, touch, orientation, and spatial awareness. The temporal lobe is associated with speech (mainly the left side) and sound, and the occipital lobe (positioned towards the back of the brain) controls sight and visual processing.

As well as the lobes, other parts of the brain control certain actions. The cerebral cortex is the outer layer of grey tissue folds that cover the brain and this is associated with the conscious movement of muscles and with processing external stimuli. The cerebellum is tucked away under the lobes, along with the brain stem. It is principally concerned with the regulation of posture, muscle tone, and muscular coordination. The corpus callosum is a band of tissue that joins the two hemispheres, allowing information, via electrical impulses, to pass back and forth between the two halves.

Although different areas of the brain are associated with particular functions, both mental and physical, none of them is able to work successfully without the complex interaction with other areas. And much of this interaction is still not fully understood, even with modern technological advances such as brain-imaging (see box on left).

MRI and PET scans

Magnetic Resonance Imaging (MRI) works by magnetizing the atomic particles present in body tissue, then bombards them with radio waves, which can be picked up by a system called Computerized Tomography (CT) and then converted into x-ray-like images.

Positron Emission Tomography (PET) produces a similar result to MRI, with a more colourful, but less defined, image. It requires the patient to have an intravenous injection of a radioactive marker, so is not particularly suitable for frequent investigations.

Both of these types of scans are used to pick up abnormalities that may occur in the brain.

The limbic system

This system is situated in the mid-brain area beneath the corpus callosum and it is not under our conscious control. It is an extensive system and includes many substructures that have their own names. Studies using modern technological advances, such as brain-imaging by PET and MRI scans (see box opposite), show that depressed people have abnormal brain activity. The frontal lobes of the brain show under activity, while areas of the middle brain, such as the amygdala (see below), become more active.

Hormonal control
The hypothalamus and pituitary gland are responsible for triggering the release of depression-related hormones such as the stress hormones noradrenaline, adrenaline, and cortisol.
The pineal gland is a small structure that begins to secrete the hormone melatonin in the evening, as daylight fades. Melatonin is implicated in Seasonal Affective Disorder (SAD; see pages 116–17).

The anterior cingulate gyrus seems to be involved in conditioning and the consciousness of self.

The midbrain is the control area of the brain, maintaining all the essential regulatory mechanisms of the body such as respiration, blood pressure, alertness, and sleep.

The mamillary body acts as a relay station, transmitting information around the brain.

Cerebellum

Brain stem

The olfactory bulbs are connected to the limbic system, helping to explain why certain smells evoke strong memories and emotional responses.

The hippocampus is key in the formation of long-term, explicit memory. Memory, particularly of trauma, is often central to depression. Stress causes the release of hormones, such as cortisol, which stop the hippocampus from working properly, leaving a person with the impression that they have been through a trauma but with no memory of the actual event.

The amygdala is a small, walnut-shaped organ that registers emotions such as fear as well as negative thoughts.

Body chemistry

To understand how the brain communicates with the rest of the nervous system it can help to think of this complex organ as a huge circuit board covered with billions of branch-like cells, which are called neurons. These neurons, which make up about 10 per cent of a brain's cells, send electrical impulses between each other to stimulate the activity in all areas of the brain and, eventually, the body.

Electrical signals

In between the branch tips of each neuron is a tiny space, called a synapse. In order for the electrical signal to pass from neuron to neuron across a synapse, to stimulate brain activity, the neuron has to release a chemical molecule called a neurotransmitter. It is thought that a deficiency of certain neurotransmitters is involved in causing depression.

Hormones

Hormone production can be disrupted for a number of reasons. Factors include illnesses (such as Cushing's syndrome, where cortisol levels are raised), thyroid problems, medication, and mood-enhancing drugs such as cocaine. Childbirth and, of course, stress can also cause changes in hormone levels.

Hormones and neurotransmitters

The endocrine system consists of a collection of hormone-producing glands. Although organs such as the pancreas, thyroid, and ovaries or testes are all part of the system, they are mainly regulated by the pituitary gland in the brain. Many of the hormones that are produced by this system are commonly associated with mood disorders.

Cortisol is a steroid hormone that is secreted by the adrenal gland. It plays a key part in the "fight or flight" mechanism (see box, top right). However, its role in depression is unclear although, where there are high levels of cortisol, the function of serotonin seems to be impaired (see box, bottom right).

DHEA, or dehydroepiandrosterone, is a hormone that is said to act on the effects of cortisol. Low levels of DHEA, along with high levels of cortisol, are found in many depressed people.

Dopamine is a neurotransmitter that acts on levels of arousal; too little dopamine is said to be a factor in depression. Low levels can also affect the control of voluntary physical movement, while high levels can cause the abnormal perceptions that are seen in schizophrenia.

Melatonin is produced by the pineal gland when the body's internal clock, situated in the hypothalamus, believes it is night-time. Those studying Seasonal Affective Disorder (SAD) think that some individuals are susceptible to the increased melatonin that is produced during the longer hours of winter darkness (see pages 116-17).

Neurons

Neurons whizz electrical impulses across the different areas of the brain to send messages to the rest of the body.

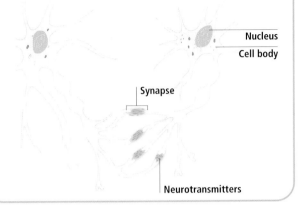

Nucleus

Cell body

Synapse

Neurotransmitters

Noradrenaline is a chemical that is associated with physical and mental excitement. Produced mainly by an area in the brain stem called the *locus coeruleus*, but also by the adrenal glands, it is involved in mood regulation. Low levels are linked to depression.

Serotonin is also known as 5-HT or 5-hydroxy tryptamine. This neurotransmitter may be familiar due to the publicity surrounding antidepressant drugs such as Prozac, which raise the serotonin levels in the brain to counteract depression. Low levels of serotonin are linked with depression, aggression, and impulsive violence whereas high levels relate to happiness and optimism.

Sex hormones such as oestrogen and testosterone are known to have a powerful effect on our moods. Contrary to popular opinion, both men and women produce both hormones in varying degrees. Pre-menstrual tension, loss of libido, menopausal problems, and postnatal depression are all thought to be partly caused by abnormal levels of these hormones.

Thyroxine is a thyroid hormone that can cause depressive symptoms if there is too little of it in the blood. An underactive thyroid can cause lethargy and weight gain. Alernatively, an overactive thyroid produces high levels of thyroxine, which, in turn, can cause agitation, tremors, and heart palpitations.

Fight or flight

The fight or flight instinct occurs when we find ourselves in stressful circumstances. For instance, imagine you have just realized your boss is leaving for the airport and you've forgotten to book her ticket. Your amygdala registers the fear and sends a message via the neurons to the hypothalamus. This then triggers the pituitary gland to release ACTH (adrenocorticotrophic hormone), which, in turn, stimulates the adrenal glands to produce adrenaline and cortisol. You will feel your heart pounding, your gut contracting, and your brain whirring. These are the results of the stress hormones flooding your body and raising your blood pressure and heart rate. It is this buzz that allows you to act quickly under such pressure.

Cortisol

Studies show that abnormally high levels of cortisol are found in up to 50% of severely depressed people. This is thought to be due to the stressful events that appear to trigger most depressive illness.

Biological contributors

There is little known about the complex interaction of brain processes in depression, but we do know more about the mechanism that makes the hormones and neurotransmitters. These chemicals cannot be created or maintained without the help of proteins, amino acids, and our genetic programming. We cannot change our genes, but we can influence our protein and amino acid levels by the food we eat.

Amino acids and proteins

Amino acids are chemical compounds that make up proteins. The body needs these proteins to maintain its overall health. There are 25 different amino acids, eight of which are known as "essential amino acids", as the body cannot function without them. These can only be obtained through the protein taken in from our diet and they include; valine, leucine, tryptophan, l-phenyl alanine, and lysine. Two of these, l-phenyl alanine and tryptophan, are needed in the production of the stress hormones serotonin and noradrenaline. They are found in foods such as meat, fish, peanuts, and sesame seeds.

Genes and depression

DNA (deoxyribonucleic acid) is the long molecule that makes up a chromosome and contains the genetic information that controls the body's growth and functioning. Each cell in the body is made up of 23 pairs of chromosomes. Genes are arranged in sequences along the lengths of DNA, and these provide the code for all our inherited characteristics.

So is there a specific gene that controls depression? Most experts agree that depression does run in families so genes are involved. But they also agree it is unlikely that any one gene is responsible. This is further complicated by the fact that it is hard to separate genetic inheritance from environmental influence. For example, if a child is brought up by a parent who is depressed, this might make the child more vulnerable, quite aside from any inherited genes. Statistics show that children with two depressed parents are said to be 50 per cent more likely to succumb to depression than those with parents who do not suffer from the illness.

Gender studies

An American study done in 1996 showed that marital status is also a factor in depression. Firstly, those with a family history of depression have up to three times higher a risk of suffering from it. Married men have lower rates than unmarried men, whereas married women are at higher risk than their unmarried counterparts. Separated and divorced people also have higher rates. There are between 10–14 million people depressed in any one year in America.

Evolution and depression

Only the fittest survive, so does the proven genetic link with depression suggest that at some stage in evolution depression had a survival value? Studies with apes showed that depressive behaviour, which is by nature passive and withdrawn, could be a survival mechanism against a superior opponent as the ape exhibiting this type of behaviour appears to be non-aggressive.

To try and separate the two contributing biological factors, to test the degree to which genes rather than the environment influence depression, research has been carried out on sets of identical and non-identical twins. Most results show that if one twin of an identical pair suffers from a depressive illness, then the chances of the other twin also suffering are twice as high as in a non-identical pair. And someone who has a parent with depression but is actually raised in a foster home is still more likely to become depressed than a child in care whose biological parents did not suffer from depression at all. For non-identical twins, the chances of the other suffering are higher than in the general population, but not as high as the chance is with identical twins. Bipolar affective disorder, or manic depression, carries an even greater genetic probability. So it seems a genetic link is indeed part of the story.

But biological links are just that, links. Although pharmaceutical companies that market antidepressants such as Prozac tend to imply that depression is an illness with solely biological causes, antidepressants are only one aspect of the treatment that can be successful in combating depression. There is a point to be made, for instance, in the high placebo response in clinical trials that test out antidepressants (see the box on page 133 for a discussion of this). The bulk of current research still suggests that the explanation for depressive illness rests in the much more complicated interaction between biology, psychology, and our social environment and conditioning.

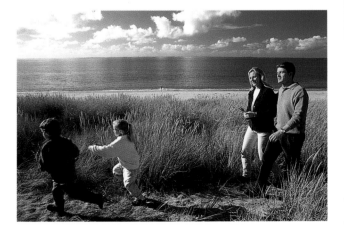

Genetic inheritance

What do we actually inherit from genes? Is it as specific as unreliable hormone production or a faulty transmission along neural pathways in the brain? Or does it merely mean that we have a predisposition to depression, given a number of other factors that have to come into play too? Unfortunately, no one yet knows the answers to these questions. One recent 10-year study carried out in Canada on the brains of people who had committed suicide discovered the presence of a gene mutation that affects a particular serotonin receptor, making less serotonin available. Another brain-imaging study showed that the brains of depressed people who had a family history of depression had one area of their brains, in the pre-frontal cortex, that was actually smaller than it should be. However groundbreaking this research is, it is not the whole story though. For instance, how do we explain the people who have these abnormalities but are not depressed or suicidal?

It seems our parents influence our predisposition to depression from the moment we are conceived, not just by the way they raise us.

Root causes

Why does one person, when faced with a traumatic life event, manage to cope and eventually move on while another sinks into a depressive illness? The answer is that we don't know, but we do understand that a number of factors are involved. The good news is that, with depressive illness so much on the increase, we are all realizing that those with depression are ordinary people who are just reacting to today's many stresses in a particular way.

The acknowledged predisposing factors in depressive illness all apparently interact with each other like a jigsaw puzzle. To get a clearer overall picture of depression we need to know what all these things are. We have already discussed the biological conditions but to these we must also add psychological factors such as early life traumas, social factors such as divorce, and medical factors.

One of the problems in identifying any of the factors that are said to cause depression is that while some people will become depressed when one particular factor is present, others will not. So to say that flu, for instance, is a cause of depression is misleading. Flu does not cause depression, but it has been seen to be a trigger in some people. It is important, however, to acknowledge that certain physical illnesses produce depressive episodes in a high percentage of people. Adversely, depression can affect the immune system, making the sufferer more vulnerable to actual physical illness. So, we must look at depression as a multi-faceted disease, and be broad-minded about the factors that contribute to the condition.

Psychological aspects

The psychoanalyst Sigmund Freud was the first to identify depression in psychoanalytical terms in his paper "Mourning and Melancholia" in 1917. He decided that depression was caused by the patient unconsciously turning his or her anger at the loss of a loved one inward. Popularly summarized as "anger turned inwards", it was the first of many psychoanalytic theories about depression.

Learned helplessness

Infant Rhesus monkeys spend their first weeks of life in close physical contact with their mothers and form an attachment bond. Even as they get older, their mothers are their secure base. Monkeys that are separated at birth and hand-reared for their first month, then placed in small social groups, are more likely to display depressive symptoms, becoming anxious and adopting a motionless foetal position.

Attachment

John Bowlby is a British psychoanalyst and is the author of the attachment theory (1981). This theory states that secure attachment to the mother is necessary for a person's future ability to separate healthily from her and form other relationships and this is thought by many to be key in depressive illness. Put simply, if a child cannot feel safe enough to separate from his mother, he risks being unable to develop a healthy sense of self, and can therefore suffer from low self-esteem and poor relationships in later life, becoming vulnerable to depression.

Helplessness

M E P Seligman (an American psychoanalyst) offers another theory (1974) that states that the grief that is felt when a loved one is lost creates a sense of helplessness. The event is beyond a person's control and so she gives up, becoming withdrawn and passive. Not every person suffering from depression will have lost a parent. But many may have had the equivalent experience in childhood with a mother figure who was unable to be there for them, for various reasons. Then, in adult life, when faced with a loss such as the death of someone close, losing a job, or experiencing failing health, the person cultivates an unconscious belief that any action is pointless and depression is the result.

Negative thought patterns

Another theory, known as the "cognitive" approach, which was actually developed separately in the 1970s by Aaron Beck and Albert Ellis (both American psychologists), suggests that it is the way we think about ourselves and our environment, more than the reality of our lives, that affects our happiness. Negative thought patterns distort the way we react to other people and life events, and create distress. Cognitive Behavioural Therapy (see pages 108-111) therefore sets out to help a person recognize the way he is thinking, test the evidence for his distorted belief blueprint, and then change the way he approaches his problems.

Distorted truth

The British psychologist Dorothy Rowe, in her classic book *Depression, The Way Out of Your Prison* (1983), also believes that depression is created internally by seeing a set of negative opinions about ourselves and our environment as absolute truths. She sitesbeliefs such as: "no matter how good and nice I appear to be, I am really bad, evil, valueless, unacceptable to myself and other people". This may mean that we believe that if we dislike ourselves then it naturally follows that others will dislike us, despite all the evidence to the contrary. This distorted "truth", Rowe suggests, can create a lifelong struggle to be "good" which, when we fail even in a small way – as we all inevitably do – will mean that we experience a terrible despair at what we see as a failure to be perfect. This, according to Rowe, is one of the cornerstones of depression.

Our internal messages

It appears then, that the distortion of our internal messages about ourselves and others is a vital component in mood disorders. And being able to understand these messages through therapies that take the cognitive approach is now recognized, in all but the most severe cases, to be one of the successful treatments for depression.

Whatever our psychological make-up, it seems we have created a society that strives to be permanently happy, rich, beautiful, and thin. Perhaps this is the legacy of not having to worry about where the next meal is coming from. But happiness for most of us is made up of moments, such as a beautiful walk, our child's embrace, or hearing your favourite piece of music, rather than being a permanent condition. If we feel that we should always be happy, or that everyone else is, then we will inevitably end up miserable as we are striving towards an impossible goal.

Belief blueprint
Negative patterns created in childhood can affect the adult life. They are established, according to Beck, early in life when we develop a blueprint for our belief in ourselves and others. So, for instance, a person is taught by her carers to believe she is unlovable and stupid. Then, in adult life, she is faced with a trauma, such as her husband running off and leaving her. She interprets the situation according to her belief blueprint and decides he has left her because she is unlovable and stupid. Beck's cognitive theory states that, although a person's thought patterns might minimize the positive and therefore magnify the problem, they are not actually beyond control.

Social factors

The social factors that might contribute to depression fall under three main headings: undue stress, isolation, and change. Again, these factors are only part of the story. There are many people who experience such problems but are not troubled by mood disorders. What is important to remember is that what may seem an insubstantial worry to you can prove overwhelming for someone else.

Public perceptions of mental illness

(from a recent American survey)

71% believe it is due to emotional weakness

65% think that it is a result of bad parenting

45% believe it is the victim's fault, and that they should be able to snap themselves out of it

43% see it as incurable

35% feel that it is the natural consequence of some sort of sinful behaviour

10% think that it has a biological basis, which involves the brain in some way

This survey shows that while some people have a little understanding, there is still a lot of ignorance and prejudice about depression. This has to be readdressed, for the sake of those suffering at the moment, and for those of us who will in the future.

Stress

The benefits of modern technology are undisputed, but wasn't life more relaxed before mobile phones, faxes, the Internet, and fast food? We do ourselves no favours by trying to live at such a busy pace as it can be a source of constant background stress.

Divorce A stressful life event such as divorce or the breakdown of a relationship is an added pressure in such a lifestyle. And it does not just affect the two people directly involved, but also the family, extended family, friends, and work colleagues. Even in the most inadequate of marriages, there is the holding pattern of status and a social network. Take that away and then mix in jealousy, rejection, loss, and feelings of failure and it is hardly surprising that going through a divorce or similar situation can trigger depression in a vulnerable person.

Bereavement The feeling when someone dies that we can never see them again, no matter what we do, often creates a sense of futility in our existence. We have very poor rituals in the Western world for acknowledging grief; so many of us try to get over a death as quickly as possible and not burden our friends and relatives with our sadness. This is not a healthy reaction and it is especially easy to open the door to depression when clamping down on unexpressed grief.

Job loss Losing a job not only removes our status and familiar daily routine, but it also separates us from our work friends and can create serious financial anxiety. Whatever the circumstances, there can often be twinges of inadequacy and panic about whether we will ever be employed again.

Poverty Being poor is extremely difficult. As well as the endless worry of how we will pay bills and clothe and feed our family, it can cause a loss of self-esteem and social status. In extreme cases it can also affect our health.

Isolation

Society is much more mobile these days, due to many different factors such as the advances in transport and the search for employment, but this has caused, to a certain extent, the breakdown of communities and the dispersal of the extended family. Many of us now live our lives surrounded by people we don't know.

There can also even be a feeling of isolation within the family; people who are at home all day with young children can feel this particularly intensely. Stepfamilies can produce feelings of isolation too, especially for the children of a previous marriage. Spiritual isolation is also more and more common these days, with church attendance at an all-time low. Without a spiritual context for our existence, it is easy to feel that there is nothing to strive for and no point to our lives.

Change

Despite the fact that change is one of the fundamentals of life, many of us find it very threatening. Rites of passage such as marriage, having children, those children leaving home, and ageing all represent types of change that can be difficult to adjust to. But, as well as these, there are changing attitudes within society at large. Male and female roles have been set in the same dynamic for centuries but nowadays men are expected to watch childbirth, change nappies, and make supper as well as work, while women are pressurized to work and still have babies, look after the home, and cook. Feelings of guilt at not being able to cope with it all are universal.

The speed of new technology is also so frightening to some of us that we become entrenched in our old ways and refuse to move with the times. The more we do this, the more we realize that we are being left behind, and the prospect of catching up can be totally paralyzing.

Stress now and then
Our modern world did not invent the word "stress". All generations have had their own versions. Ours often stems from pollution and the pressure of endless communication. But go back as far as prehistoric man, when there was not a machine in sight. They had the stress of survival: if they didn't catch their supper they couldn't eat. Whatever form it takes, there has been, and always will be, stress in humans' lives.

Being aware
We are all prey to some or all of the social and environmental situations that have been described on these pages at different times in our life. Experiencing such pressures does not mean that we will necessarily fall immediately into depression. But if a number of these factors are present at any one time, or we are in a susceptible state when one or two occur, they can be the nudge that sends us spiralling into depression. It is worth being aware that this can happen – both for ourselves and for those around us with whom we interact closely.

Physical causes

There are certain medical conditions that can produce symptoms of depression in those affected. But although diseases that directly affect the brain can actually cause a depressive episode, most that are linked with depression are merely catalysts – not all the people who suffer from them will succumb to depression. Chronic illness and other factors such as allergies can also trigger depression.

Rehab programmes

A Finnish study done at the University of Central Hospital in Helsinki in 1998 found that three months after release from hospital, 54% of first-time stroke survivors not enrolled in rehab programmes, which included social activities and support, were depressed. This was a higher figure than those who attended the programmes; only 41% of these people suffered from depression.

Multiple Sclerosis

It is said that 10% of Multiple Sclerosis sufferers are also affected by depression as they are prone to mood swings. No one is clear why this should be, although the degeneration of the myelin sheath – the fatty layer that protects nerve fibres in the brain and the spinal cord – means that the body's electrical circuitry is damaged. This reduces the electrical impulses that travel to and from the brain and body.

Head injuries and stroke

Accidents occurring to the left side of the brain, whether it be a brain haemorrhage caused by stroke, head injury, or tumour, are particularly associated with depression. This is thought to be because the right side of the brain, associated with the emotions, is no longer being controlled by the injured left side, so emotions run riot. Right brain injuries can have the opposite effect, making the affected person unrealistically optimistic.

Diseases and suffering pain

In Parkinson's disease, the dopamine-producing cells no longer function properly, so the levels of the neurotransmitter dopamine are lowered. Too little dopamine affects the sufferer's ability to move voluntarily, induces muscle tremor, and is linked to depressive symptoms such as low moods and lethargy.

Diseases that do not affect the brain directly, but which are frequently linked to depression, include glandular fever, hepatitis, flu, and ME (myalgic encephalomyelitis). No one knows why depression sometimes follows these viral illnesses.

Many diseases of the endocrine glands also affect depression. Cushing's syndrome causes an excess of the hormone cortisol, which is said to reduce the efficiency of the neurotransmitter serotonin. Up to 50 per cent of people with this disease experience depression. Thyroid malfunction is also implicated in depressive symptoms. Excess of the principle thyroid hormone, thyroxine, produces anxiety and palpitations. Low levels, known as hypothyroidism or myxoedema, cause lethargy and mood dysfunction and can present themselves as depression.

People who suffer from a chronic illness such as rheumatoid arthritis also seem to be vulnerable to depression. No organic link to brain malfunction has been established in these cases, but it is hardly surprising that ongoing disability through illness that is little understood can make the sufferer depressed. Other diseases, such as cancer, can cause high anxiety levels associated with the fear of death (see box, top right). It also doesn't take much imagination to accept that someone suffering from chronic pain might lapse into depression. Pain is very tiring, mentally and physically, and so the many of us who suffer from extreme migraines or back pain can also become depressed.

Other causes

Vitamin and mineral deficiency If we are depressed we may not eat properly. In turn, certain vitamin and mineral deficiencies can make us feel depressed (see pages 56–9).

Allergies There is also some evidence that sensitivity to substances such as wheat and sugar can trigger depression, although this area is under-researched at the present time.

Medications Prescription drugs given to treat other diseases can sometimes be linked to depression. For example Reserpine, which is used to alleviate high blood pressure, reduces serotonin function and causes depression in up to 30 per cent of recipients.

Alcohol Excessive alcohol consumption is a common cause of depression. It reduces the activity of certain neurons in the brain and this state is often found in depressed people (see page 50).

Lack of sunlight Light deprivation can cause a mood dysfunction known as Seasonal Affective Disorder. It is thought that the reduced hours of daylight in the winter months cause the pineal gland to produce too much melatonin, the hormone that helps us to sleep, causing lethargy and depression (see pages 116–17).

So many things have been listed here that you may conclude that anything can be a contributory factor. But remember that it is the interaction of a range of these things that causes a person to be depressed. And the specific factors are different for everyone.

Terminal illness
Many people diagnosed with a terminal illness go through depression before accepting their approaching death. There are five recognized stages of dying:
Denial: it can't happen to me.
Anger: life isn't fair – why me?
Bargaining: just let me live until my grandchild is born…
Depression: I can't bear this, but there is nothing I can do.
Acceptance: I'm ready to die, it doesn't frighten me anymore.

Aspartame
There is new evidence that the artificial sweetener Aspartame may reduce the levels of serotonin in the brain, leading to mood and sleep disturbances (see box on page 50). Taking large amounts may result in headaches, nausea, memory loss, and depression.

Seeking help

Most of us are terrified to admit to any sort of weakness that relates to our psychological state. We would more comfortably confess to something like bowel cancer than depression. This may be because our psychological function is inseparable from our psyche – how we think and feel about ourselves is who we are – whereas parts of our body can be put at a safer distance from our feelings and be treated in a more mechanical way. Mental dysfunction, therefore, strikes at the root of our self-perception and often scares us. And because this unspoken fear has now evolved into a social stigma, many of us affected will not ask for help, even from our closest companions.

Another block to avenues of help is the fact that, as we said earlier, depression often has an ill-defined beginning. It can come on almost overnight, or can slowly evolve over weeks. Most of us experience mood fluctuations that render us temporarily low, as well as periods of low energy. Therefore it can be difficult for those of us affected to recognize when a low mood actually impacts on our work or relationship seriously enough to be considered as depression. It is often hard to decide when it is time to seek help.

It may be necessary for those around us to point out that we have a problem, and this first step has to be followed by an acceptance on the part of the depressed person before any sort of action can actually be taken. If we do accept that we need help, we must then identify what kind of help would suit us as an individual, and from whom we can best obtain it.

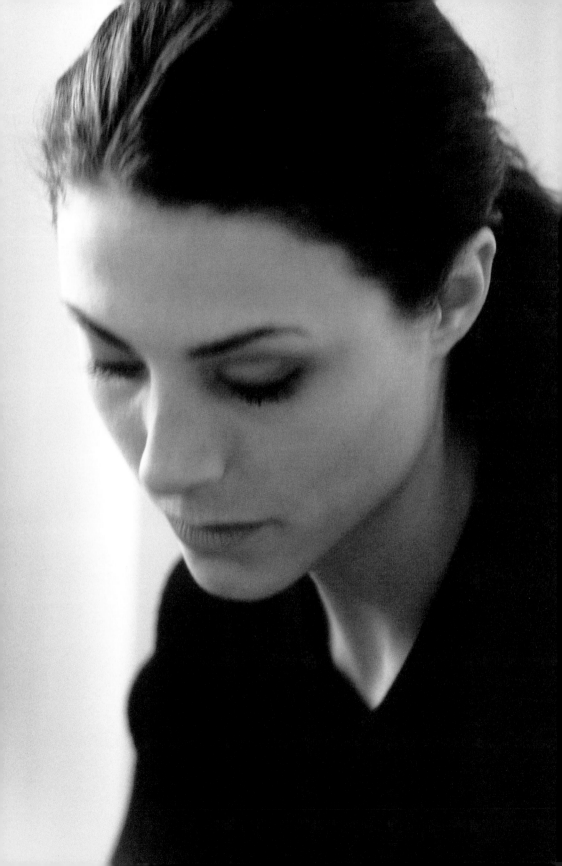

When to seek help

One of the most difficult problems with depression is knowing when to seek help. It is often hard to be objective about our own moods, and to focus on how we are feeling with enough clarity to realize the degree to which we are depressed. We know we aren't feeling right, but we gloss over the fact that our low mood has been going on for a long time and is beginning to affect those around us too.

Signs to look for
- Have any of your family or colleagues commented regularly on your moods or suggested you have problems?
- Have you felt unusually disinclined to engage with those you are close to?
- Is your partner complaining that you no longer want a sexual relationship?
- Have you noticed that things you used to do with ease now seem either frightening or overwhelmingly difficult?
- Do you feel generally like running away, hiding in bed, or doing something destructive?
- Have you lost interest in your general appearance?

If you can say yes to three or more of the above, and these have occurred over a period of a few weeks, then it would be sensible for you to seek some professional help.

Who to go to

Doctors are concerned with our bodily health, and this is inextricably linked with our mental health, so it makes sense that the local doctor's surgery should be the first port of call if you realize you need help. This also means that they should be able to eliminate the possibility of symptoms having a physical, rather than a mental, cause. In an ideal world a doctor will listen to the patient and then find out any background history, such as stressful events or life changes. Depending on the symptoms, he or she will then give a physical examination, check blood pressure, and may also take blood for testing. A course of treatment will then be advised, based on the assessment, or another specialist will be called upon for their opinion too.

However, this ideal scenario may not be the reality that you experience. This could be due to the fact that the symptoms of depression can be very easily masked by physical problems. For instance, you may go to a surgery complaining of sleeplessness. It is easy for an over-worked doctor to hurry along without really listening, and to send you off with a pat on the back and a packet of sleeping pills. Or the doctor might listen long enough to register that you are depressed, but have no time to assess the degree of the condition, and no knowledge, money, or facilities to offer anything but a course of antidepressants. In the UK, for instance, Cognitive Behavioural Therapy on the National Health Service is hard to come by and the sessions are usually offered only once a month anyway. Luckily, more and more surgeries are taking on counsellors and other therapists of their own, so it might be worth finding a practice that has these added facilities if you find out that yours hasn't got them.

What to say To make the most of an appointment, it is important to give as much information as possible to a doctor. You shouldn't be embarrassed or ashamed, as you have as much right to ask for help with depression as you do for, say, a stomach ulcer. Try to be as honest as possible, even if your thoughts are painful, because otherwise your doctor will find it difficult to help you. You will also feel much better when you have spoken up. Making a list of symptoms, stating how long they have lasted, and what you are feeling about yourself, is a good thing to do before visiting your doctor. It also sometimes helps to get a close friend or relative to tell you how they see your general moods and behaviour.

If the doctor diagnoses depression and then prescribes you with antidepressants, you should also ask what alternative treatments the practice offers that could be taken either instead of, or to supplement, the medication. These might include herbal medicine, homeopathy, or acupuncture. The doctor may also be able to recommend a local therapist.

Complementary and alternative therapies refer to treatment systems other than those employed in conventional medicine. If a complementary or alternative therapy is decided upon, there are many associations and registers that will ensure that you find a qualified practitioner. It will probably mean that you have to pay for the treatment, but the levels of payment vary and are often negotiable. "Ways to improve your mood", on pages 44–155, describes, in much more detail, some of the therapies that can be used to combat depression.

Someone to listen What we all need, above everything else, is someone who will really listen to what we say. If you don't feel up to explaining how you feel to a doctor, or don't feel able to ask the appropriate questions, then you should take someone along who you know is capable of doing it for you. If, however, you do go on your own and, when there, sense you are not being listened to and are being fobbed off with medication you don't really want to take, then you should ask to see another doctor in the practice, or return with additional support and insist that you get a re-evaluation.

Public perceptions

The medical journal the *Lancet* reported in October 1999 that after the "Defeat Depression" campaign in 1998 by the Royal College of GPs and the Royal College of Psychiatrists in Great Britain, the public now view counselling and psychotherapy as the most beneficial types of treatment, more so than antidepressant drugs that were once thought to be addictive.

Treatment options

Finding the right treatment option is often the biggest problem when we are depressed, because we are probably not in the mood to initiate ideas, question the doctor's decision, or take in details about each medication. However, it is vital to know the pros and cons of what every avenue of help is really offering. And we must also remember that there are alternatives to medications too.

Drug dependency

Dependency, or addiction, occurs when the physical or psychological comfort of a person depends on regular use of a drug. This means that there will be a need to increase the amount of the drug to get the same level of comfort and the person will not be able to stop taking the drug suddenly without experiencing prolonged withdrawal effects.

Medications

There are three types of drug associated with the treatment of depression: tricyclics, monoamine oxidase inhibitors (MAOIs), and selective serotonin reuptake inhibitors (SSRIs). Valium, a drug from a different group called benzodiazepines (which are used for anxiety and insomnia), was often prescribed to depressed women in the 1960s and 1970s and thus became known as "mother's little helper". It is no longer popular as it can create dependency if used over long periods, and does not have antidepressant action. Antidepressants, however, do not cause dependency.

Tricyclics When neurotransmitters such as noradrenaline and serotonin are released into the brain, they are usually quickly taken up again into the cells. These drugs block this process, thus increasing the levels of the two neurotransmitters that are available to stimulate the brain. Some tricyclics, such as amitriptyline (brand name Tryptizol), also have a sedative effect, and can be used if insomnia and anxiety form part of the depression. However, side effects such as dry mouth, blurred vision, sweating, and constipation are common.

Monoamine oxidase inhibitors (MAOIs)

These are usually given if tricyclics are not working, or the person also has problems with anxiety or phobias. They work by blocking the action of the enzyme monoamine oxidase, which normally breaks down the neurotransmitters, and this results in raised levels of neurotransmitters to stimulate the brain. MAOIs are used with great caution because of their dangerous interaction with many medications and foods, which can create potentially life-threatening reactions. People taking these drugs must avoid many cold remedies, as well as tyramine-containing foods such as cheese, red wine, and yeast extract.

Selective serotonin reuptake inhibitors (SSRIs)

These drugs block the reuptake of the neurotransmitter serotonin. More serotonin means increased brain stimulation. Fluoxetine, brand name Prozac, and paroxetine, brand name Seroxat, are the most popular. Although they have fewer side effects than the tricyclics, SSRIs can produce insomnia, anxiety, nausea, and headaches in some people. Recently the pharmaceutical industry produced modified versions of SSRIs, with drugs that affect both serotonin and noradrenaline.

Tricyclics, MAOIs, and SSRIs take effect two to six weeks after beginning the course. The length of time they are taken varies according to the severity of the depression and how well a person responds to the drug. Research has shown that they must be taken for at least six months once a person has responded to that drug in order to prevent a relapse.

Talking therapies

Therapies such as counselling and interpersonal therapy focus on our childhood and past experiences. Cognitive Behavioural Therapy works to change our thought processes while Cognitive Analytical Therapy combines both these disciplines. Sessions are usually given at least once a week and last for 50 minutes, which is known as the "therapeutic hour".

Complementary and alternative therapies

These therapies include physical disciplines such as yoga and Tai chi as well as mental exercises such as meditation, hypnotherapy, and visualization. Changing nutritional intake will also help to enhance moods and improve brain function. There are also spiritual disciplines and therapies that work on the senses, such as aromatherapy, light therapy, and massage. The big advantage of alternative therapies for those who are depressed is that a vital part of each of these treatments is listening and relating to the whole person – the holistic approach – rather than just treating the individual symptoms. Details of all these therapies are given on pages 64–155.

Electroconvulsive therapy (ECT)

This is a controversial therapy that was overused in the past and is now only viewed as a last resort treatment. A patient is given a general anaesthetic and muscle relaxant, then an electric current is administered via electrodes applied to their forehead. It isn't yet known exactly how the therapy works, but it appears that the electrical current causes the patient to fit and this creates change in the chemicals in the brain. This therapy can alleviate severe depression, particularly psychotic depression, but the side effects include short-term memory loss, confusion, and headaches. There is also the risk of the anaesthetic to consider when using this treatment.

Ways to improve your mood

Feeding
your mind

Eating healthily, research now insists, makes us feel better and function more efficiently while protecting us from disease. So the now familiar mantra of "more fruit, vegetables, and fibre, less fat and sugar," should be taken seriously by us all.

But the relationship between food and depression is, as with all areas of the illness, difficult to define. Eating a nourishing diet is not necessarily going to prevent depression, particularly if there is a strong psychological basis to the illness. Neither does consuming mostly sausages, chips, and Coke automatically bring about a depressive episode. There are certain foods, however, which can directly affect our mood and food sensitivities are also now considered to be a trigger of depression.

One of the problems with depression is that we often change our eating patterns for the worse. We skip meals, comfort eat with too much of the wrong sort of food, take in too many toxins, such as alcohol and nicotine, or are inclined to consume junk food because it provides a quick sugar high. As a result, our body does not get the right nutrients and we can easily become vitamin deficient, which then exacerbates any low moods we are suffering from. We may also become overweight, which will further affect our self-esteem.

Balancing our diet, regulating our meals, recognizing food sensitivities, and avoiding toxins are all ways to keep healthy. But we should also consider the role vitamins, minerals, and herbs, as well as supplements, can play in our physical and mental well-being.

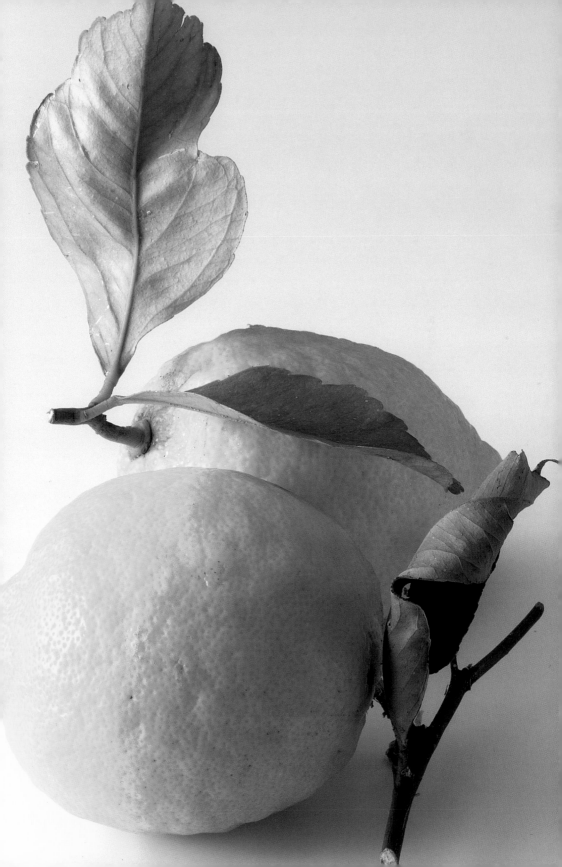

Do you know how to balance your diet properly?

Do you crave sugary foods regularly during the day?

Do you have to have a drink to relax?

Food for thought

We are all different, and our personal nutritional needs vary according to many factors – from genes to environmental conditions – but there are sensible, general guidelines that we should all try to follow. To keep our bodies and minds in tip-top condition, we need 50 essential nutrients each day, and we can only get these from the food that we eat.

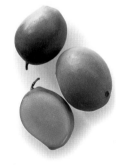

It is far better to eat plenty of fruit than to overdose on meat.

Hints and tips

Steam your vegetables.

Cook vegetables whole, then slice them afterwards. This helps to retain more nutrients.

Eat food as fresh as possible, and from a source that has a frequent turnover so you know it hasn't been lying around.

Frozen food has better nutritional value than old or poorly stored food.

Tasty, colourful food will help to stimulate the senses.

Food types

Our food is divided into types, and consuming the right percentage of each, every day, is what keeps us healthy. But don't panic, it is not an exact science. It is important that you enjoy your food, especially if you are suffering from depression.

Carbohydrates There are two types of carbohydrate: sugars and starches. Sugars found in fruit and vegetables are natural, or slow-releasing – they release sugar slowly into the bloodstream. Those found in sugar, cakes, biscuits etc are refined, or fast-releasing – they supply a sudden burst of sugar into the bloodstream. Starches found in plant foods such as wholegrain rice, wholemeal pasta and bread, and potatoes are known as complex, or slow-releasing, carbohydrates. These are high in fibre, which fills us up and is essential for a healthy digestive system. Refined, or fast-releasing, starches are found in pasta and bread made from white flour, as well as in white rice, but these do not enable the body to work as efficiently.

Refined sugars, such as cakes and biscuits, are implicated in mood swings. They give us a fast energy buzz as our blood sugar level rises, but equally quickly they produce an energy low because the sudden increase of sugar in the blood sets off a reaction from the hormone insulin, which absorbs the sugar into the cells so the blood sugar levels slump. Therefore we eat a biscuit for example, feel energized, then feel tired again, so we eat another biscuit and so on. It is much better to eat an oatcake with hommos, or a couple of pieces of dried fruit if we want a much more sustained, healthy energy boost.

Proteins Made up of 25 amino acids, proteins are essential for making hormones and neurotransmitters, as well as for the healthy growth and development of our bodies. The best sources are fish, beans, lentils, meat, soya, and eggs. Because these foods contain the amino acids trytophan and l-phenyl alanine, which make serotonin, they help to keep us happy. But the brain can only use a certain amount of these amino acids, and most experts agree that we eat too much protein, especially animal protein, which is more difficult to absorb. Excess protein is just excreted and wasted – it is much better to eat more fruit.

Fats There are two types of fat, saturated and unsaturated. Saturated fat is the sort we get from dairy products and meat, and it is usually solid at room temperature. Unsaturated fat is either polyunsaturated, found in vegetable, sunflower-seed, fish, and nut oils, or monounsaturated, which is found in olive and rapeseed oils. A recent American study has shown that eating high levels of certain polyunsaturates known as omega-3 and omega-6 fatty acids, mostly found in oily fish such as salmon, mackerel, and tuna, is linked to lowering levels of depression.

Water The body loses more than 1.5 litres (2¾ pints) of water a day through breathing, sweating, and urinating, which needs replacing. Coffee and tea are not advisable alternatives because of the toxins they contain. More importantly, caffeine causes diuresis – it makes us urinate – and therefore also tends to dehydrate our bodies.

Getting the most from our food

How we select, store, and cook our food has a direct bearing on the amount of nutrients we get from it. All those vegetables and fruits that we are always encouraged to eat are only as good as the soil they were grown in. They are also affected by the levels of pesticide spray they have been subjected to, which is why the organic alternatives are gaining in popularity. The length of time before food reaches the shops and the way it is stored also affects it. Boiling food, for instance, loses up to 50% of its nutrients. If it only had 50% to start with, then the benefits will be almost non-existent.

Nutritional amounts

Carbohydrates are our main body fuel and the complex, unrefined sort should make up 50–70% of our daily diet.
Protein should make up only 10–15% of our diet.
Fats, preferably unsaturated, should form 15% of our diet.
Water is lost from our bodies constantly so we should drink at least 1.5 litres of water a day to top up our fluid levels.

Eating three portions of oily fish every week is good for our brain as well as our body.

Sabotaging nutrition

The nutrients the brain needs are often sabotaged, particularly during depression, by unhelpful toxins such as alcohol and caffeine. We tend to use these substances because they give us a temporary lift but, when we are depressed, there is a tendency to overuse them. Food and chemical sensitivity can also unbalance our body chemistry, causing depression in some people. There are some who consider a high percentage of depression to be caused by such food sensitivities.

Alcohol and depression Alcohol is confusing. The first glass or two acts as a stimulant and we feel relaxed, brighter, and more at ease. But alcohol is actually a sedative and depressant, so a low mood always follows the initial high. This results in us having to have another drink to feel better, and then another. Some of us actually drink excessively without realizing it.

Alcohol leaches important vitamins, particularly the B group and vitamin C, from the body. It is true, however, that red wine in moderation provides antioxidants – the chemicals that mop up cell-damaging free radicals in the body. But heavy drinkers are usually poor eaters so they end up depleting their body's

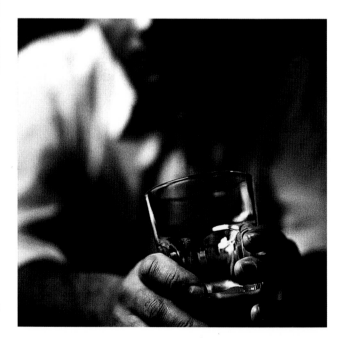

Too much alcohol, as we all know, causes wide-ranging damage to our minds and bodies, especially if we are regularly using it to escape reality.

nutrients. In general, alcohol worsens sleep patterns, causes mood disturbances, anxiety, and depression, and will interfere with antidepressant medication. And it kills off brain cells.

Caffeine and depression The caffeine in coffee and tea interferes with the absorption of important vitamins. And, like alcohol, caffeine produces an initial burst of energy followed by a low mood, which creates a need for more caffeine. If we consume more than three cups of tea or coffee a day we are actually exceeding the recommended amounts of caffeine and may experience caffeine toxicity. This results in shaking, increased heart rate, lowering of the body temperature, mood disturbance, anxiety, irritability, and disturbed sleep.

Food sensitivity Although this is a relatively new area of research, there is some evidence to show that some people become depressed because they are eating a food that they are sensitive to. The reason for this reaction is not clear. British nutrition expert, John Briffa, thinks it may be due to inadequately digested food leaking into the bloodstream. This food, instead of generating energy, interferes with normal metabolism. Foods associated with allergies are dairy products, the gluten in wheat, and, to a lesser extent, rye, oats, and barley. Although we have been eating wheat and drinking milk for centuries, the sort of wheat we now eat and the way today's milk is produced and treated is thought to be to blame. It is best to see a nutritionist if you think you may have a food sensitivity.

Sugar intolerance and our guts We've discussed the fact that sugars can be mood disrupters, but if a person is actually glucose intolerant they will crave excessive amounts of sweet and starchy foods. When they eat these foods, however, too much insulin is released into the body, making their blood sugar level drop hugely. This is known as hypoglycaemia, and can cause symptoms such as tiredness, dizziness, irritability, palpitations, and depression.

Blood sugar balance can be checked with a blood test and any imbalance rectified by reducing sugar, coffee, tea, and alcohol, eating a wholefood diet, and using vitamin/mineral supplements. Always go to a qualified nutritionist or doctor for this treatment.

Candida
Our gut needs a proper balance of bacteria in order to function properly. If we eat a poor diet, take antibiotics, or are on the Pill, the balance of a fungus called candida can be upset. It is particularly sensitive to sugar, even the type found in fruit. Candida is said to be a contributory factor in many illnesses, including depression.

Test your diet first
If your depression has a predominantly psychological basis, then nutrition therapy is not going to help, although it will ensure you are eating a nutritious diet. But it is worth considering having tests for biochemical imbalance and food sensitivities as part of the diagnostic process before deciding to take medication.

Has eating stopped being a pleasurable experience?

Do you often skip breakfast because you are too busy?

Is your diet boring and unvaried?

Good mood foods

A good appetite is usually a sign of a healthy digestive system. Most of us would probably complain that our appetites are rather too good! But that might not actually be true. What often happens is that we respond to the huge number of "eat, eat" messages that continuously bombard us through advertising and convenient, fast-food outlets. Consider this question: are you really hungry each time you eat?

Food strategy

Eat what you like, not what those around you want you to.

Eat breakfast. Your blood sugar levels are low at this time.

Snack on fruit and wholefood as often as you want. This keeps your blood sugar balanced.

Buy colourful food that looks fresh and tempting.

Don't cook if you don't want to. Eat a salad, some cheese and fruit, and/or a piece of fresh brown bread.

Have nutritious "fast food" handy, such as avocados.

Eat a variety of foods so that you don't get bored.

Indulge occasionally without feeling guilty.

Don't be tied to meal times. You are much less likely to overeat if you know you can have a snack in an hour's time.

Eat slowly and savour your food – sit down to eat it.

When we become depressed, often the first physical sign is an altered appetite. Food loses its pleasure for us, and we often have to force ourselves to eat anything at all. Or else we eat and eat to try to fill the hole of our unhappiness, rather than to quench an appetite. However, we do need strategies to help us eat as well as possible even when we are not feeling like it.

Foods to enhance our mood

We have already discussed the way carbohydrates and proteins act directly on the production of serotonin and noradrenaline in the brain to lift our moods. But the B vitamins are also implicated in brain and nerve function and mental health.

The B vitamins There are five B vitamins, which work best together. They are not stored in the body, so it is important that we have a regular, daily intake of them in our diet. Vitamins B3 and B6 are involved in the manufacture of tryptophan, the amino acid that makes the neurotransmitters serotonin and noradrenaline. You might be familiar with the names of the B vitamins from reading the side of cereal packets (see box, right).

Vitamin C This vitamin is important for various reasons. Firstly, it is essential for a healthy immune system, which is usually poor in depressed people. It also helps to make anti-stress hormones and is an antioxidant, fighting the cell-damaging free radicals we take in via stress and pollution. It is also vital for the absorption of iron into the system. If we lack sufficient quantities of iron we become anaemic, which in turn will make us depressed. Vitamin C cannot be stored in the body, so we must keep up a daily intake from the foods we eat. Good sources include oranges and lemons, kiwi fruit, peppers, tomatoes, and broccoli.

Food is energy When we are experiencing a low mood state we often have no energy. So it is vital that we get as much help as possible from the food we eat. If you are used to eating large quantities of cakes and pastries, sugar, and meat without any fruit, vegetables, and fibre, then it's going to take time to change your habits. But it is surprising how much better you will feel when you do. Our bodies respond quickly to a healthy diet, and soon your body will tell you that it needs more fruit, green vegetables, or a glass of fresh juice. There is no need to rush for the brown rice. Go gently – begin by replacing a sugary pudding with creamy yoghurt and fresh fruit, add a few more vegetables to your plate of meat, and cut out one of your daily coffees. By doing these things you will have already increased your essential nutrients, and therefore your body's overall energy levels too.

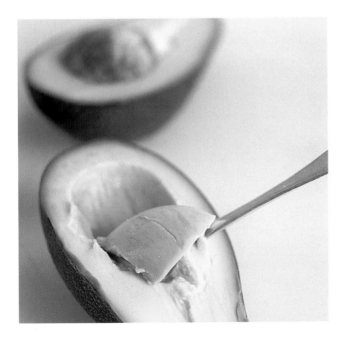

The B vitamins
Thiamin, B1, is essential for brain function. Good sources include watercress, enriched breakfast cereals, and beans. **Riboflavin**, B2, metabolizes fats, sugars, and protein. Good sources are mackerel and broccoli. **Niacin**, B3, is good for energy production and brain function. Sources include tuna and chicken. **Pyridoxine**, B6, is essential for hormone production and brain function. It is also a natural antidepressant. Sources are bananas, peppers, and nuts. **Cyanocobalmin**, B12, is good for the nervous system. Good sources for this vitamin include sardines, eggs, and cheese.

Enzymes explained
Enzymes are the chemical substances that break down the food we eat so that it can be absorbed by the body. Raw food increases your enzyme levels because it contains high quantities of enzymes that become active during chewing, getting digestion off to a good start. When it's cold and miserable we feel low, and raw food is not appealing. But an apple, a banana, or chopped up vegetables with a dip are worth trying when we feel like this as they will make a difference.

Next time you fancy a fast-food snack, why not try half an avocado with a squeeze of lemon.

Do you suffer from bloating after you have eaten?

Do you think your low mood could be related to your diet?

Are you prone to asthma or eczema?

Nutrition therapy

With the increasing awareness of food sensitivities, it makes sense, if you are feeling depressed, to check that you are not suffering from any food allergies. A nutrition therapist treats disease with diet and nutritional supplements rather than drugs. Although it has long been understood that diet can affect health it is only recently that nutritional medicine has become an accepted alternative therapy.

Testimonial

Sarah had suffered a series of emotional shocks, but four to six weeks later she started getting physical symptoms such as hyperventilating, tiredness, ballooning weight, depression, and what is known as "brain fog" – she just couldn't think or string a sentence together. She even felt suicidal. She saw doctors and psychologists, but to no avail, then an alternative therapist suggested that she should try excluding wheat from her diet. Within two days all her symptoms had vanished.

What does a nutritionist do?

At your first appointment you will be asked lots of general questions about your health and medical history, and the symptoms that have been particularly bothering you. The nutritionist will want to know things like how much alcohol and coffee you drink, if you smoke, whether you exercise, and if you are taking any medication. She/he might examine your nails, eyes, and tongue, as all these can show up signs of nutrient deficiencies. Some nutritionists will also take blood, sweat, and hair samples to test in a laboratory for a more detailed run down of your body's biochemistry. Or they may do the more sophisticated IgG ELISA (enzyme-linked immunoserological assay), which tests for sensitivity to more than 50 foods.

Depending on your symptoms, you will probably be asked to keep a food diary for a week or two. This will require you to write down everything you eat and drink and describe how it makes you feel. For instance, if you have a sensitivity to wheat you might feel bloated when you have eaten a plate of pasta. On your next visit you will be given a personal diet sheet that tells you which foods to eat and which to avoid. You might also be given a vitamin, mineral, or herbal supplement. Re-educating ourselves regarding the way that we eat can be difficult, and results are not always instant. Some people actually feel worse before they feel better, as the body adjusts to the changes in the diet and detoxifies itself. You might also find family meals tiresome if you can't eat what everyone else is eating. But persevere, and be honest with your therapist. If it isn't working, say so. Often the initially rigorous diet can be modified quite quickly. For instance, if a mild food sensitivity is diagnosed, you may only have to stay off that food for between two and six months before reintroducing it gradually. You may also only have to see your nutritionist as little as three times – obviously this will be more often if the problem is not responding to treatment.

Why choose a nutritionist? As the symptoms of depression are often as physical as they are psychological in kind – ie we experience palpitations and dizziness along with low moods and lack of self-esteem – it can be difficult to identify when the cause is linked solely to a biochemical reaction such as food or chemical sensitivity. It is worth considering this possibility before starting a long-term drug therapy, especially if you have eczema, asthma, allergies, drastic mood swings, or digestive problems.

Learning about nutrition and focusing on the way we eat can have a lifetime benefit. As we get older and our bodies are more susceptible to diseases brought about by poor nutrition, we can help ourselves to live a longer, healthier, and happier life. There is definitely a connection between longevity and decreased calorific intake – the less we eat, the longer we live!

Hints and tips

If you have been checked for food sensitivities and have found that this is not actually the root of your problem, it is still worth following some of the tips below, even if you only try one or two of them. Don't get into checking the size of the portions you eat, or try to eat stuff you don't like just because it's healthy. And don't punish yourself if you have a day when you only eat rubbish.

Consume wholefood rather than refined food.

Eat lots of fruit and vegetables every day, some of them raw.

Take in lots of foods containing B group and C vitamins.

Eat food as fresh as possible.

Make sure that you eat little and often.

Drink plenty of pure water.

Avoid too much alcohol as well as tea and coffee.

Don't feel guilty if you give in to the odd indulgence.

Be aware of the possibility of food sensitivity.

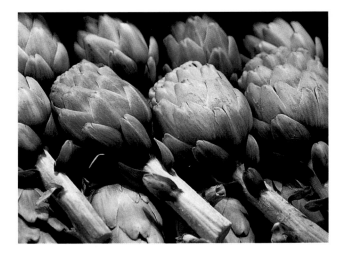

Make your diet more exciting by introducing lots of variety and tasting things you haven't tried before.

Are you getting enough vitamins from your food?

Do you view supplements as unnatural and unnecessary?

Is food the last thing on your mind?

Vitamins and minerals

Whether or not we need to support our diet with vitamin, mineral, herbal, or hormonal supplements is a debate that rumbles on between the professionals. There are more and more messages in the media telling us to take supplements to make us younger, stronger, and, happier. In the end it all sounds a bit baffling – is there any supplement that helps depression? Or is there one that might prevent it altogether?

Guidelines

- Get the bulk of your nutrients from food, not supplements.
- If you are depressed and are not eating properly then take a multi-vitamin supplement with adequate levels of B group vitamins, and extra vitamin C.
- Don't take supplements singly without professional advice – they work better synergistically.
- We all have different needs. If you are in any doubt about what is best for you, then consult a nutritionist first.

Getting what we need

The RDA, or recommended daily allowance, is the benchmark, set by World Health Organization doctors and scientists, by which we are told to monitor our nutrient intake. But these levels are in fact set at disease-prevention levels, not for optimum health. For instance, the RDA for vitamin C is 60mg, whereas most research suggests that 400–1000mg are necessary to make any real difference. However, despite the fact that the RDA levels are set to prevent diseases like rickets (lack of vitamin D) and scurvy (lack of vitamin C), rather than to improve our general health, there are large quantities of the Western world's population who don't even manage to obtain these low levels of nutrients on a daily basis.

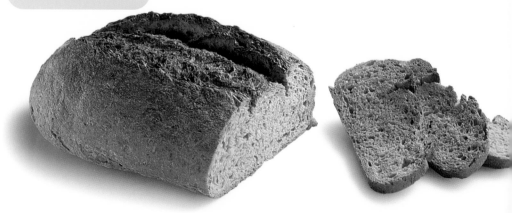

The next point to consider is that we are all different. Whether we eat healthily or not, our health is also affected by our genetics, environment, age, economic status, and whether we are ill, pregnant, or on a restricted diet. So the RDA can only be a very general guideline.

Taking vitamin and mineral supplements

Vitamins and minerals work synergistically – they only work, or work best, alongside another nutrient. So taking an iron supplement when your vitamin C levels are very low will minimize the supplement's effect as vitamin C aids in the absorption of iron. On top of this, iron supplements interfere with the absorption of zinc, so if you are taking iron it is wise to take zinc too.

Why do we need supplements? Should we be taking these supplements at all? Why can't we just eat the nutrients we need and forget about supplements, except in the case of an illness based on a specific nutritional lack, such as iron-deficiency anaemia? Well, in an ideal world we could get all the nutrients we need from our food, but most of us don't. If you have a good daily balance of properly cooked, fresh, pesticide-free food, live in an unpolluted environment, are happy and stress-free, and are in good health, then you probably won't need supplementation. But most of us have good days and bad days with our food. Days when we forget lunch because we are too busy, drink too much coffee, or go out drinking in the evening and grab a late-night pizza. Every day, for most of us, is not a five-portions-of-fruit-and-vegetables day. So, particularly if we are depressed and food is the last thing on our mind, it makes sense to give ourselves the best possible chance of optimum health, by taking a multi-vitamin and mineral supplement, with sufficient levels of the B vitamin group to help keep our mood up, and vitamin C to strengthen the immune system and encourage the production of anti-stress hormones.

Although there is no such thing as an anti-depression vitamin, there is enough evidence to show that a body receiving a good nutritional balance will have the best chance of fighting off disease, and certain vitamins, such as the B group and C, can directly affect our moods.

Getting a balance

Why can't we just take vitamins and mineral supplements instead of food, especially when we don't feel like eating?

The experts do all agree that getting the bulk of your nutrients from food is better than eating a poor diet and relying on supplements, because the right food contains the whole balance of fibre, protein, fats, and calories, whereas the vitamin pill only delivers the vitamin.

No one quite knows if vitamins are as effective in pill form as they are when absorbed directly from food.

We can't overdose on vitamins and minerals very easily from food, unless we are eating an extremely restrictive and obsessive diet. But, for example, if you take too much vitamin C in supplement form (the amount will vary depending on your age, weight, and overall health) then you could suffer from diarrhoea.

Supplements ought to be considered as just that, supplements, and not the main source of our daily nutrients (see pages 61–3 for a discussion of other supplements that can help depression).

Wholefood carbohydrates, as found in brown bread, are much healthier than their white counterparts, so stay off the white sliced loaf.

Do you find that you get ill at regular intervals?

Do you worry about what supplements to take?

Do you eat enough oily fish?

Taking supplements

There is so much difference of opinion about what vitamin and mineral supplements to take, and how much is needed to be effective, that it has to be down to each individual to decide whether to supplement their diet or not. But by taking a general consensus of studies, the following guidelines (if you do choose to take supplements) will give you an idea about what and how much is likely to be both safe and effective.

Vitamin toxicity

Many of us worry that supplements can actually damage our health. And it's true that overdoses of vitamins can cause some side affects (see box, top right). However, it must be stressed that vitamin and mineral toxicity is very rare, and if you follow the guidelines on the vitamin bottles, or stick with a standard, high quality multi-vitamin, you should not have any problems of this kind.

Vitamin C

This vitamin is also known as ascorbic acid and the RDA is 60mg. There have probably been more debates about vitamin C than about any other supplement in the past few years. Opinions vary about exactly how valuable high doses are in treating diseases like cancer, heart disease, osteoarthritis, and the common cold. But enough research exists to merit taking at least 1000mg a day, either in fizzy tablets, slow release capsules, or powder form. These work better when taken alongside bioflavonoids, the antioxidants found in fruit and vegetables. Too low a level of this vitamin will affect your moods because it assists in the making of anti-stress hormones and neurotransmitters, as well as working to strengthen the immune system. You would have to eat a vast amount of vitamin C-containing fruit to obtain the optimum levels, so taking a supplement does make sense.

B vitamins

This group includes the vitamins B1, B2, B3, B5, B6, and B12. Do not take any of these vitamins separately as they work better together – high doses of a single one can cause side effects (see box, top right). The best vitamin B supplement is a B complex supplement, or a multi-vitamin pill that includes B vitamins. This vitamin group is essential for brain and nerve function and the alleviation of mood swings so higher levels can help depression.

Omega-3 and omega-6 oils

Known as essential fatty acids (EFAs), alpha-linolenic acid and linoleic acid are important for brain and nervous system function. One research study showed that women with a high intake of omega-3 (alpha-linolenic acid) had lower levels of depression. Opinion varies as to what ratio these two oils should be taken in. Flax seed oil is rich in both, but has a higher percentage of omega-3. So it is advisable to take one tablespoon of flax seed oil a day – or a high-dose fish oil capsule (1000mg) containing two other EFAs, EPA (eicosapentaenoic acid) and DHA (docosahexaenoic acid). Alternatively, eat three portions of oily fish (mackerel, salmon, or tuna) per week.

Potassium

Lack of this mineral can make a person feel low, and usually comes about if that person has been taking diuretics for some time, or has had a long bout of diarrhoea. Potassium helps in insulin secretion, which regulates the blood sugar and keeps our moods stable. Potassium works with sodium in the body, so if you have had a bad stomach upset with vomiting and diarrhoea, a rehydration drink consisting of ½–1 teaspoon of glucose and a pinch of salt dissolved in 100ml (3fl oz) of hot water should help to rebalance your potassium levels. Alternatively, try eating a banana or some garlic.

Magnesium

This mineral is important for the functioning of the nervous system and energy production. Again it is better not to take it alone, but as part of a multi-vitamin and multi-mineral supplement. Or you could eat some Brazil nuts or sunflower seeds along with it.

Folic acid

Low levels of this vitamin have been positively linked in some trials with depressive symptoms. It is thought that a folic acid deficiency interferes with the body's ability to make serotonin and dopamine so it is important to keep the levels up. It is found in foods such as yeast extract and spinach, and works best alongside the B complex vitamins. A therapeutic supplement dose for adults is between 400 and 1000mcg a day.

Side effects

These are not common but you should still be aware of them.

Vitamin C: very high doses can have a laxative effect.

B vitamins: B3 and B6 taken alone in high doses can cause nerve and liver damage.

Omega-3 and -6: if you are on blood-thinning medications, or are pregnant, too much of these oils will hinder blood clotting.

Potassium: high doses are toxic.

Magnesium: more than 1000mg a day can cause flushing, low blood pressure, and breathing problems.

Folic acid: more than 15mg can produce gastro-intestinal upset and sleep problems.

Daily doses

Taking more than the recommended doses of any of these supplements in an attempt to either prevent depression, or make it go away, will not work and will only put you at risk of toxicity, so please don't try it. It is definitely best to obtain your vitamins and minerals from fresh food rather than supplements. However, if you are depressed or are just not feeling at your best, it is sensible to supplement your diet with a good quality multi-vitamin and multi-mineral supplement, and a daily dose of 1000–3000mg of vitamin C, which can be obtained from a health-food store.

Do you sometimes feel anxious or panicky?

Do you feel in desperate need of a tonic?

Do you forget things quite regularly?

Botanical remedies

Herbs have long been recognized for their healing properties in the traditions of Chinese and Ayurvedic (Indian) medicine, but the West has been slow to catch on, despite the fact that many conventional drugs are the synthetic version of ingredients in medicinal plants. But how can we get the most from plants and are there actually any natural alternatives to conventional antidepressants?

Hints and tips

Plants can be as potent as any conventional drug, and the current sentimentality about anything "natural" must not make us blind to the possibility of side effects and toxicity of inappropriate herbal application. Despite the fact that popular depression remedies such as St John's Wort are available over the counter, it is always advisable to consult a doctor or herbal practitioner about your symptoms first.

And if you are worried about the dosage or suitability of any of these medicinal supplements, then consult a nutritionist or herbalist before using them.

Culinary herbs

Cooking with herbs is a simple and safe way to gain benefit from the many wonderful healing properties they contain. They can be dried, infused in oil or in water for tea, or eaten fresh on salads and in sauces.

Borage *(Borago officinalis)* A plant of Mediterranean origin, borage is called the "herb of gladness", as it is said to lift the spirits, steady the nerves, and relieve anxiety. Use it in salads.

Lemon balm *(Melissa officinalis)* This refreshing herb has calming properties and helps the digestive system when it is upset due to anxiety. Infuse it to make tea, or use it in salads or cold drinks.

Parsley *(Petroselinum crispum)* Rich in iron, vitamin C, and carotenoids (health-giving plant chemicals), parsley is good for the nervous system and can help anxiety and mild depression. Sprinkle it on soups and salads or make it into a sauce.

Rosemary *(Rosmarinus officinalis)* Rosemary is associated with love and remembrance (see yellow box, right). Its blood-stimulating properties are said to aid memory and help with migraine and depression. Infuse it in some oil and add a few drops to a bath or bake it with lamb, chicken, or fish.

Sage (*Salvia officinalis*) The Greeks thought that sage made them live longer, but it is also good as a tonic for the nerves and helps memory and poor concentration. It is delicious with duck, in stuffing and omelettes, or with pasta.

Plant supplements

Plant supplements have become increasingly popular as aids for our general health. However, a few of them are also significant in the treatment of depression.

Gingko biloba This is an ancient species of tree and its leaves have been used in the East to enhance memory for thousands of years. It stimulates the blood supply to the brain, improving the overall function. Supplements of Gingko biloba can be taken in tablet or capsule form, and it is best to find one that has a 24 per cent flavonoid concentration. The recommended dosage is 80–160mg per day, divided into three doses. It can take at least a month, probably more, before any improvement is noticed.

Ginseng There are two main types of this supplement: *Panax ginseng* (Asian ginseng) and *Eleutherococcus senticosus* (Siberian ginseng). Called "adaptogens" – substances that strengthen the body's ability to fight stress and restore hormonal balance – both are excellent tonics for those who are run down.

Panax ginseng is seen as an overall rejuvenator of mind and body. Taken in recommended doses (normally 100mg of ginseng extract twice daily), side effects are uncommon. But it is not advised for those with high blood pressure, anxiety attacks, manic depression, or for pregnant women.

Eleutherococcus senticosus is thought to be a good tonic for those who are tired and stressed. Take 180–360mg a day in two or three divided doses.

Milk thistle (*Silybum marianum*) This detoxifies the liver and protects it from the damage caused by pollutants, drugs, and alcohol. It is also good for those who are on antidepressants and is an antioxidant. Take 160mg three times a day but, if you have liver damage, consult your doctor before using it.

Cold infused oil

This recipe can be used for massage, bath oil, or inhalations: take a sterilized storage jar and pack it with your herb. Cover this with almond oil and seal it with an airtight lid. Leave the jar in a sunny place for two weeks, shaking it daily. Then open it and squeeze the oil through a muslin bag into a jug. Pour this into sterilized, dark-coloured, airtight storage bottles and then label them and put them aside for later use.

"There's rosemary, that's for remembrance. Pray you, love, remember. And there is pansies, that's for thoughts."
Hamlet, Act 1V, scene V

Herbs are not only health-giving – they smell wonderful and are a great addition to the kitchen and the bathroom.

These pretty, yellow flowers that belong to the St John's Wort plant are the source of a popular and effective therapy for mild or moderate depression.

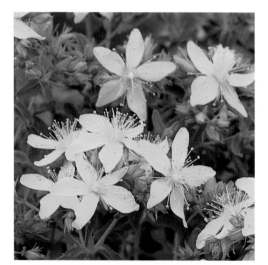

Herbal supplements as antidepressants

The plant substances already mentioned are important in supporting the body and mood when a person is depressed, or to help prevent the likelihood of a depressive episode. However, there are also a few herbal supplements, namely St John's Wort, 5-HTP, and Kava, which are used as alternatives to prescription drug treatments. St John's Wort is Germany's leading anti-depressant drug, accounting for over 50 per cent of the market.

St John's Wort (*Hypericum perforatum*) This is thought to be called St John's Wort because its yellow flowers appear around the saint's day on June 20th. The whole plant is used for the dried extract. The active ingredient is thought to be hyperforin. Although there has been extensive research into the plant, which proves its efficacy in treating mild and moderate depression and SAD, no one is entirely clear how it works.

Hypericum raises levels of the three main neurotransmitters – serotonin, noradrenaline, and dopamine – in the brain, aids sleep, and acts as an anti-anxiety drug. It takes at least two to six weeks to be effective, and, most importantly, the side effects (headaches and dizziness) are mild and rare. Recent reports have suggested that St John's Wort increases sensitivity to sunlight, with one American study warning that hypericum can react with ultra-violet light to damage the proteins in the eye, possibly causing cataracts. But there have been no reported cases of hypericum-induced cataracts, and it is thought the doses would have to be exceptionally high to make this a worry. However, health authorities in the US are also warning that there are new suggestions that it can raise blood pressure, reduce the effectiveness of low-dose oral contraceptives, and react badly with some dietary supplements. But these recent concerns can be combated by the millions of people who have used this drug over the past two decades. There have been no reports of serious toxicity at all, even when it has been taken in large doses. It is also non-addictive and does not cause cognitive malfunctions. Measure all this against the very real and unpleasant side effects of prescription drugs for depression, and you can see why St John's Wort has become so popular.

There is a need for caution when using St John's Wort, though. As it is available over the counter, some people take it when their problem is not actually depression. It is always wise to see your doctor for a diagnosis of your symptoms first, even if you then choose St John's Wort instead of a prescribed medication. For the dosage it is best that you consult your doctor and read the leaflet that comes with the product you buy.

5-http (5-hydroxytryptophan) This comes from the plant *Griffonia simplifica* and raises the serotonin levels in the brain by increasing levels of tryptophan. Studies show it to be as effective as the SSRI drugs and no side effects have been recorded so far.

Kava Kava (*Piper methysticum*) Kava belongs to the pepper tree family and is native to the South Pacific islands. The root produces the active ingredient, kavalactones, which South Pacificans make into a drink. This has been found to be an excellent treatment for relieving anxiety, insomnia, and lifting moods, although research has not yet shown how it works. One theory is that it affects the amygdala, an area of the brain that deals with emotional responses (see pages 24–5).

Kava is now approved as an effective natural tranquillizer for the treatment of mild to moderate depression, anxiety disorders, and phobias. Side effects are minimal and rare if taken in the approved dosage, which varies depending on the percentage of kava extract in the capsules. It also comes in tincture and powder forms. As with St John's Wort, consult your pharmacist for a suggested dosage.

Valerian (*Valeriana officinalis*) Depression plays havoc with sleep patterns and Valerian can aid natural sleep. It is, however, less effective than synthetic pills for short-term, acute insomnia, as it can take a week or two to have an effect. It is best taken one hour before bedtime. Lower doses can be taken to reduce anxiety and stress and side effects are rare.

Conventional vs natural

It would be foolish to suggest that there is no place for conventional drug treatment in depression. But, despite the growing appeal of natural medicines, there is still a prevailing wisdom in some countries that "natural" is somehow New Agey, and therefore not as effective as prescription medication. Now, especially with the extensive trials of alternative medication that have been carried out, this attitude is looking much more outdated.

Although many do not suffer from the sometimes terrible side effects of antidepressants like Prozac, plenty of others do. It seems sensible, therefore, to try out the natural alternatives that have been proven to have minimal problems, before embarking on the much more toxic, synthetic versions.

Get advice

It is best to consult your doctor before using any sort of herbal supplement, as you need to be aware if the herbal preparation you have chosen will potentially interact with any conventional medication that you are taking. Remember the rule that you should always treat any substance you take into your body with respect.

Have you recently been through a traumatic experience?

Do you often feel tense in your throat or stomach?

Do you generally lack self-confidence?

Flower remedies

Flower essences have been used for healing for thousands of years. The Australian Aborigines and Egyptians were among the first practitioners of flower therapy. Useful for mild depression, these remedies are gentle, working with the sufferer to calm and restore when they are distressed. Sessions with a flower essence therapist can also help to shed light on the emotional pattern that might be at the root of depression.

How it works

Severe stress of any kind creates an imbalance in our energy systems, making us both physically and emotionally vulnerable. Practitioners of flower essences believe that the energy patterns in flowers correspond to our own subtle energy and can be utilized to bring our systems back into balance and so free the body up to heal itself. Specific flowers relate to certain psychological and emotional states – for instance, the flower Star of Bethlehem acts on psychic trauma and shock to produce calmness and serenity.

How flower remedies were developed

We owe our modern system of remedies to Dr Edward Bach, a respected doctor and homeopath, who developed his 38 remedies in London, England in the 1920s. He decided that harmful and negative emotions, and how different personality types respond to these emotions, were at the root of all disease. He then looked for a healing system within the plants and flowers in the fields around London. In recent years there have been many other essences developed, which have been inspired by Dr Bach's system, from places like California, Hawaii, and the Australian bush.

Dr Bach obtained his essences by picking the blooms of fresh, wild flowers and floating them in bowls of spring water left in the sun for two to three hours. The tincture this produced was then preserved in brandy at a ratio of 50 per cent brandy to 50 per cent flower water and stored in a dark glass bottle.

How to take flower remedies

Bach developed his healing system to be applied by the patient, either by deciding what his or her emotional state was and then taking the appropriate essence, or by dowsing. Dowsing involves using a crystal on a chain or piece of string as a pendulum; it is held over each remedy and when the right one is found the pendulum swings round in a circle. It is also common for a practitioner to work with a patient, examining their symptoms to find the most helpful essence, or group of essences, for them as an individual.

To take the essences, dilute the concentrated solution with spring water and drop them under your tongue, or, alternatively, drink them from a glass. Doses vary from four to ten drops of the concentrate, which can be taken three or four times a day, or more frequently in acute situations. You can also apply the drops directly to the skin – the best places are the lips, wrists, forehead, and palms. Alternatively, just add a few drops of flower essence to a warm bath. There are no known side effects when taking these flower remedies.

Rescue remedy The most famous of Dr Bach's remedies is his Rescue Remedy. This is for emergencies, when a person experiences shock, panic, hysteria, or desperation. It is a compound of five essences: Star of Bethlehem, impatiens, clematis, rock rose, and cherry plum, and it can be taken at frequent intervals until the person finds some relief. If you are experiencing a low mood it can be helpful to carry Rescue Remedy around with you so that you can take it straight away if you suddenly feel overwhelmed.

Flower therapists A therapist who works with flower essences is experienced in the wide variety of remedies from all over the world, not just Dr Bach's. If you are not confident about your ability to diagnose yourself, it can help to work with such a therapist to select the best essences for your particular problem. One visit, with a follow-up after the essences have had time to work, is usually sufficient, although it can also be an ongoing therapy if desired.

The safety of flower essences Because flower remedies work with a person by gently tuning in to his or her energy systems, and any change is quite gradual, they are safe for anyone to take, regardless of age, and do not interfere with any other treatment. They are therefore particularly good for anyone who is nervous about the potential side effects of therapies.

Evidence

There is no scientific research to back up the effectiveness of flower remedies, but, despite this lack of evidence, Bach and other flower remedies have a wide following. Some think the beneficial effects spring from what is known as the "placebo effect", ie the person taking the drops believes they will help, so they do. But the many who have found relief in the remedies over the years say that there is a lot more going on than mere wish-fulfilment.

What flower remedies are used for

Pine is a Bach remedy for guilt and self-reproach.
Larch is a Bach remedy for lack of self-confidence.
Penstemon is a Californian remedy for self-pity or those who are feeling persecuted.
Walnut is a Bach remedy for those wishing to break away from old behaviour patterns and embrace a new way.
Olive is a Bach remedy for those tired out by long struggle.
Sweet Chestnut is a Bach remedy for unbearable anguish.
Dandelion is a Californian remedy for those with an excess of bodily tension.

Do you feel weary, lacking the energy to go on?

Do you often feel sad and upset for no reason?

Have you lost your vital urge for life?

Homeopathic remedies

Homeopathy, like flower essences, works to rebalance and vitalize our energy force. Dr Samuel Hahnemann was the 18th-century German doctor who rediscovered the healing system that has actually been around since the time of the ancient Greeks. It is now one of the most popular alternative therapies used by people today to alleviate all sorts of symptoms.

How it works

The "vital force" or energy flow that keeps us healthy becomes deformed when we suffer a physical or mental trauma. Homeopathy sees the symptoms of disease as a sign that the body is using its self-healing abilities to respond to the trauma. Homeopathic medicine is said to stimulate the vital force to concentrate its energies on the traumatized part of the body to help heal it.

Homeopathic remedies actually induce a reaction similar to the disease symptom in order to produce relief. This is known as the "law of similars". For instance, Hahnemann discovered that quinine, made from the bark of the cinchona tree and used to treat malaria, actually triggered malaria-like symptoms when given to a healthy person.

How homeopathic remedies are created

Homeopathic remedies contain minuscule, almost negligible, amounts of the particular active substance chosen for the treatment, which has been serially diluted many times with a mixture of alcohol and water, leaving hardly more than the molecular imprint of the ingredient. This is then dropped onto tiny lactose tablets. Dr Hahnemann discovered that the more he diluted a substance – a process called potentization – the more effective it was and the less likely to produce side effects.

Homeopathic treatment

It is possible to treat ourselves at home with homeopathic remedies, particularly if we are only suffering from minor ailments. Arnica, for instance, is a superb remedy for shock and trauma. If you are depressed, however, it might be wise to seek out a qualified homeopath, who will be trained to find the exact remedy to address your problem from a huge range of variants. Part of this process, for instance, involves deciding on your personality type, which can help you to understand how you might react to stress. You might, for example, be *Arsenicum album* (arsenic): sensitive, vain, creative, and well dressed, this type may seem anxious and exhausted by the world. Or you could be *Pulsatilla* (windflower): this type is highly emotional, timid, and weepy.

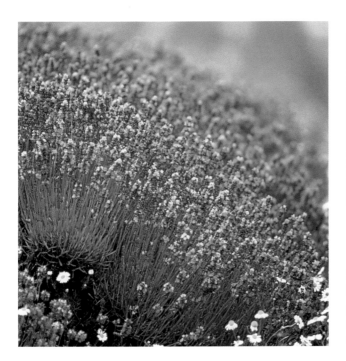

Remedies suitable for depression

Sepia is for loss of general libido, sadness, and weariness.

Natrum mur is for the stoical sufferer as well as for any form of loss or distress.

Ignatia is also effective for loss and sadness.

Kali phos is for anxiety, phobias, and emotional upset.

Material for homeopathic remedies is found in animal, mineral and plant extracts, and is roughly chopped or ground before water and alcohol is added.

Evidence

A study of migraines at the Glasgow Homeopathic Hospital in the UK in 1997 showed an interesting result. A 55-year-old male suffered from acute migraines with vomiting for three years, and these were not alleviated by conventional medicine. He took Bronia homeopathic remedy for three weeks and was still headache-free three years later.

Looking at the whole person Homeopaths use the holistic approach, treating the person as a whole, rather than just the disease. So a practitioner will ask you about your emotional state, your worries, and your lifestyle, as well as your medical history. The remedies they then prescribe are not for depression *per se*, but for the person who has presented with the symptoms of depression. So the remedy you are given for depression might be quite different from the remedy someone else is prescribed, depending on what symptoms are present.

It is important for a homeopath to get a full picture, so be prepared to explore how you feel and how the remedies are affecting you, either for better or for worse. This isn't always easy for people new to homeopathy, as the homeopath will want to know everything, from a fleeting headache to a serious pain in your gut, or if you feel weepy listening to music.

The first consultation will be at least an hour; subsequent ones are shorter. The length of treatment and number of consultations vary – sometimes a person can actually feel worse to start with, as the body adjusts to the remedy, but this does not last long.

Relax your
body and mind

As we've said before, mind and body act in unison. For our brain and emotions to function at their best, our bodies must also be fit. The problem is that the word "fit" conjures up all sorts of daunting images of super-slim people with immaculate bodies. It is easy to feel that our chances of ever looking like that are non-existent so we decide that there is no point in trying at all. But there are many different kinds of physical discipline that can relax us, make us more mobile, strengthen our hearts, and lift our spirits, without necessarily involving leotards and gyms. And the good news is that the results can be felt almost immediately; you will feel better about yourself after just one session of brisk exercise. The secret is in the brain chemicals known as endorphins, which make us feel happier and more confident. When the body temperature rises during exercise, endorphins are released and our mood improves.

But bodily movement is also more fundamental; spiritual traditions such as Ayurveda believe that movement is life, and that physical immobility results in spiritual immobility and disease, because we become disconnected from *spanda*, which is the spark of energy that allows us to be joyful and spontaneous. This makes sense if we relate such thinking to depression. When all we want to do is sit scrunched up without moving it is hardly surprising that our energy has a hard time flowing round our bodies.But we also need to balance the exercise that stimulates and releases our energy with techniques that will calm and relax us.

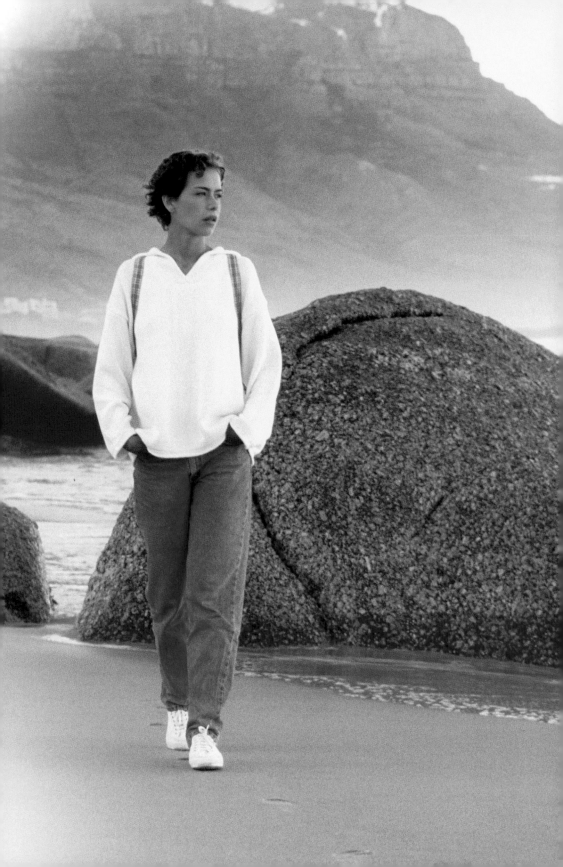

Do you feel like you never have any energy?

Do you regularly suffer from stress?

Do you find that you get out of breath quickly?

Physical exercise

For those of us trying to beat low moods, there is nothing more important than exercise. Without wishing to sound bossy, we really have got to get our bodies moving. But forget the word "exercise" for the moment, and concentrate on "movement" instead. We will look at disciplines such as yoga, breathing and relaxation techniques, and Tai chi later on, but let's start with the basics here.

How it works

Exercise makes us breathe more deeply and so raises our heart rate and the circulation of blood round our body. This, in turn, increases the supply of vital oxygen to the cells in the brain, muscles, and other organs so improving their overall function.

Exercise also helps to burn off the stress hormones, such as adrenaline, that build up when we are stressed or depressed. The endorphins that are released when we exercise actually elevate our mood and generally make us feel better about ourselves.

Getting moving

Often when we are depressed, we hold our bodies stiffly and take shallow breaths. It can be quite difficult to straighten up, let the muscles loosen, and allow our bodies to open up. But we will certainly feel better afterwards if we are prepared to take the initial risk to exercise.

One of the biggest problems with exercise is our perception of it. We think that it involves expending large amounts of energy and also necessitates organizing venues, scheduling classes, paying money, and allocating time we are sure we can't afford. So some of us will have to "trick" ourselves into getting started. We will have to pretend that we aren't actually exercising, and try a gentle form such as a quick swim to begin with. From then on the benefits of feeling more energetic will keep us going.

Find an exercise you like Exercise, like everything else we do, is a very personal thing. You might have a friend who swears by four-hour bike rides every weekend, or hour-long aerobic classes to loud music. This is obviously fine for him or her, but this doesn't mean you have to do the same thing. Most exercise regimes fail because we are not really suited to them. Think about what you enjoy. Do you like being with other people? Do you enjoy the outdoors? Do you find it easier to be in a class or to work from a book or video? Do you like team sports or games such as tennis and golf? Are you prepared to spend money on exercising and do you have the time and inclination to travel some distance to get involved in a particular activity?

Make a list and identify the factors that are important to you. You may hate classes, have limited resources, but need company to spur you on. In which case taking regular walks with a friend might be your ideal exercise.

Start small Don't rush off and join a class, or a gym, unless you've done it before and it works for you. If you're one of those people who are "allergic" to exercise, begin with something simple like a walk (see box, right). You can then gradually build up your exercise. Increase the time by five minutes, walk a bit faster so that you are breathing harder, but are not out of breath. Do an extra day each week. Very soon you will begin to miss your walk if you don't do it, and you will find that you can go further and longer without getting out of breath. Even if this is all the exercise you ever do, it will make you fitter, happier, and healthier. Wear sensible shoes, drink lots of water, and wear layers so that you can strip them off when you get warmer.

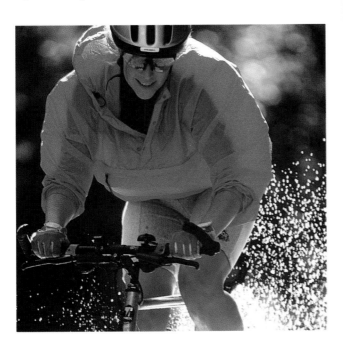

Be realistic

It is not good, particularly if we are depressed or not feeling at our best, to be too ambitious when planning what exercise to do. If you have a heavy work schedule then there is no point in booking long classes in your lunch break that are hard to get to and require changing and showering afterwards. Nor is it sensible to book a personal trainer for 6am if you can't stand getting up early. Within a week or two you will have given up and just increased your overriding sense of failure and uselessness.

Try walking

Wherever you live there is somewhere to walk, even if it is only to the next bus stop. And walking is free! It also has the advantage of being in the fresh air and sunlight. Make your first walks just 10 minutes every other day. Look around you, breathe deeply, swing your arms, and turn your face up to the sun. Have a goal such as reaching a particular shop, post box, junction, or tree and then stick to it – don't try to do any more. It may also help to try to take your exercise at the same time of day each time.

The sheer exhilaration that physical movement brings about will help to lift you out of your low mood and make you feel better about life.

Choice of exercise

It is important to find an exercise that you feel comfortable with, however low key it is, as this will make it easier to ensure that it becomes a part of your everyday life. And when you have begun to build your fitness and confidence up, you can try a more ambitious regime. But don't be press-ganged into a type of exercise that does not suit you just because it is fashionable or your best friend is doing it. While you are beginning to decide on the type of exercise that is right for you, it is helpful to know more about what exercise is and what it does. There are two main types; aerobic and anaerobic.

Aerobic exercise increases the efficiency of our heart and lungs so that they will supply plenty of oxygen to the rest of the body and brain during any activity. If we are unfit aerobically we will get puffed out doing things like climbing stairs, walking fast, or going uphill. Our hearts will pound in our chests, we'll get red in the face, and will gasp for breath when we attempt any serious exertion. Exercise that improves our aerobic fitness includes jogging, swimming, fast walking, dancing, cycling, and skipping done for sustained periods of 12 minutes or more. This is the best sort of exercise when we are feeling low because we notice the effect on our mood very quickly as endorphins are released.

Anaerobic exercise works directly on our muscle strength but doesn't involve a sustained supply of oxygen to the muscles. Examples of this include using the equipment in a gym to work the different groups of muscles in our body or doing exercise techniques such as Pilates, which uses repetitious action on each muscle group to build strength and flexibility. Although this form of exercise is important for general fitness, don't expect to see results immediately. It takes at least five weeks of regular anaerobic exercise to change the shape of our bodies.

Body image

Eating disorders such as anorexia and bulimia are often discussed these days. But there are many more of us who, while not actually suffering from these distressing diseases, have no confidence in the way we look. When we are depressed,

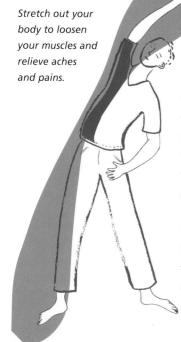

Stretch out your body to loosen your muscles and relieve aches and pains.

this problem can be exacerbated, and our eating patterns, as we discussed earlier, can go awry and induce weight gain or weight loss, which further upsets our self-image. Surveys invariably show that people, especially women, are rarely happy with the way they look.

Exercise can help our self-image enormously in many different ways. It improves our posture, so we stand straighter and taller to face the world. It also increases energy, so we're not always tired. It reduces muscle flabbiness, so what flesh we do have is firm and toned and it also burns calories, so that we are less likely to put on weight. It helps us to become flexible too, so we can, for instance, tie our shoelaces or get in and out of a car without feeling as if we are 100 years old. And the resulting improved muscle strength and mobility means that we won't suffer from the aches and pains in our backs, necks, and legs that can make us tense and bad-tempered.

The psychological benefits

There is a "smug" factor to exercise. It is seen by most of us as being a sort of virtue. We proudly tell people how many lengths we swam or how far we walked. This must be the result of being part of a leisured society, because people in countries where exercise involves picking crops or carrying water certainly won't feel the same need to boast about it. But, ridiculous as it may be, the truth is that we often see people who exercise as more functioning and successful than those who don't.

There is also a genuine sense of personal achievement in seeing our bodies become stronger and more flexible. If we haven't exercised for some time, it will seem impossible that we will ever be able to run up a hill without keeling over. But if we persevere we soon realize that we can walk up it at a pace, then we can run part of the way, and finally we can make it all the way up and are still able to breathe! Accomplishing this sort of goal makes us feel that we can conquer the world too.

Although exercise will not transform us overnight into Wonder Woman or Superman, it is a vital component in the maintenance of both our physical and emotional well-being.

Evidence
The Cooper Institute in Dallas, Texas, USA, is currently conducting a three-year research project with 120 people to see if exercise is effective in treating mild or moderate depression. They are using people between 20 and 45 who are experiencing depressive symptoms such as low moods, sleeping problems, feelings of worthlessness etc who can exercise up to five times a week at the institute.

Expending energy also increases energy and vitality, so wake up your body with some vigorous exercise and you will soon begin to feel less tired.

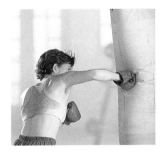

Do you feel tired all the time?

Do you know how to switch off and relax?

Does your mind race uncomfortably?

Breathing

Each one of us breathes all the time – if we didn't, we would die. But most of us are not consciously aware of how we breathe, or how important the correct breathing technique can be to our mental and physical health. Ancient Chinese and Indian healing traditions have always linked breath with our life energy, and believe that by breathing properly we can calm our minds and bodies and help ourselves to relax.

How it works

When we breathe air into our lungs the tiny air sacs within them, called alveoli, pass oxygen into the bloodstream and take back the waste product, carbon dioxide, which we then breathe out.

If we are breathing inefficiently, the balance of oxygen and carbon dioxide in the body becomes upset. Too little oxygen to the brain can make us tired and lethargic, reducing our alertness and the body's ability to metabolize food into energy. And carbon dioxide and other waste products will not be properly eliminated from the body. Alternatively, too little carbon dioxide, which is caused by over-breathing when we are tense or stressed, can lead to fainting, palpitations, and aching muscles.

Take a deep breath

Our brains require huge amounts of oxygen, more than any other organ in the body, because the neurons in the brain have a high rate of metabolism. When we deny our brain its proper quota of oxygen, we find we lose concentration, yawn, and feel tired, and can become moody and stressed. For an example of this, just picture yourself in the last session of the afternoon at university. You've been hunched over your desk in a stuffy room for hours and nothing the lecturer says goes in; you yawn, fidget, and feel irritable because your brain isn't getting enough oxygen, and carbon dioxide is building up in your body. But when you finally get outside and run for the bus, you feel energized at once and are ready to find something to do.

Most of us do not make the best use of our breathing capacity. This is because of poor posture and too much time sitting at office desks, in the car, or slumped in front of the television. Instead of using the whole of our lungs, we tend to shallow breathe with the top part only. By doing this we also increase tension in the muscles of our neck and shoulders, and this can result in headaches.

When we are depressed, our whole body metabolism slows down and all we feel like doing is curling up in a corner. This produces a vicious circle, as the more we slump in our low moods the less we breathe properly, and the less deeply we breathe the less oxygen our brains get, so the more lethargic and depressed we will become.

Stand up One of the simplest things you can do to aid proper breathing is to stand up straight. Gently pull your shoulders back and drop them, straightening the spine by imagining a cord is attached to the top of your head and it is pulling you up. By doing this your lungs now stand a better chance of getting all the oxygen that they need.

Sit up No one is saying that you can't sit comfortably in a chair and relax, but try to sit with you back supported at the base of the spine and keep your spine straight at all times. If you are eating a meal, or are sitting at your computer, don't slump. Sitting or standing up straight when we are not used to it can feel very uncomfortable at first, because the muscles in our backs have become lazy and weak. But persevere, as poor posture will inevitably cause back problems in the end, especially as you get older.

Exercise Any form of aerobic exercise makes us breathe more deeply and expands our lungs. Going for a brisk walk in the morning will help your concentration at work, or you could, alternatively, nip out at lunch for a quick reviver in the middle of the day.

Energy and breathing

Prana is the name given by Indian yogis to the vital life energy that flows through the body. They do not believe that *prana* purely refers to breath, but do feel that the two are closely connected. American holistic healer Rudolph Ballentine describes the connection as similar to us and our shadows. Yogis compare *prana* to a kite, our breath being the string that holds it, and the wind being the universal power. They say that by practising yogic breathing we can free up the energies within our bodies to help us heal ourselves and others (see box on page 77).

Evidence
Ongoing research conducted by American Dr Herbert Benson since the 1970s at the mind/body medical institute at Harvard finds that relaxation techniques, when they are combined with exercise and nutrition, are beneficial in reducing stress and anxiety.

O_2 CO_2

Fill your brain and body with energizing oxygen by standing tall and taking big, deep breaths.

Full yogic breathing or pranayama

This breathing technique, which is also recognized as the scientific technique of breath control, is said to clear and calm the mind as well as strengthen and cleanse the body. Be conscious of your breath, but let it flow; don't try to control it too much. Practise this every day for 15 minutes in a quiet place if you can.

1 Sit cross-legged on the floor, on a cushion if you like.
2 Place your left hand on your abdomen and your right on your rib cage or diaphragm.
3 Inhale through your nose, keeping your mouth closed.
4 Draw the breath slowly down into your abdomen, so that your stomach area expands first.
5 Then draw the breath upwards to feel the rib cage expand.
6 Lastly breathe into the top part of your lungs.
7 Exhale, allowing the air to leave your stomach first, then the midriff, and your upper lungs last.

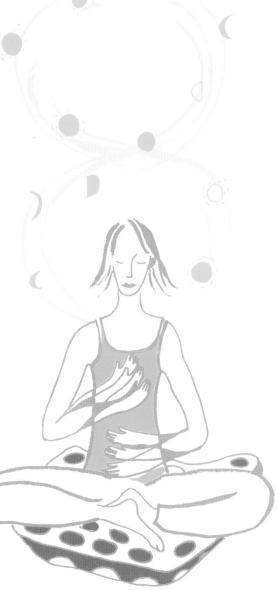

Diaphragmatic breathing

If done correctly, this method can relax your body and release tension to produce tranquillity and calm.

1 Lie comfortably on your back on the floor. A blanket or rug will make this easier.
2 Place your left hand on your abdomen, and the right on your rib cage or diaphragm.
3 Close your mouth and breathe through your nose.
4 Inhale without too much effort (your breath should not be forced or deep), allowing your rib cage to expand gently, but holding your lower abdominal muscles firm so that your stomach area doesn't swell up.
5 Exhale, allowing your diaphragm to fall naturally.

This exercise can also be done sitting cross-legged. Practise it every day for at least 10 minutes until it becomes more natural. When you are anxious it is a wonderful way to induce calm.

Cleansing breath

Called *kapalabhati*, this exercise is said to be the most effective in cleansing the body of impurities through the exhaled breath, and giving an oxygen boost to the body and brain on the inhaled one.

1 Sit cross-legged comfortably on the floor, with your hands on your knees.
2 Contract your stomach muscles sharply to breathe out forcefully through your nose.
3 Allow the breath to come back into the lungs without effort, again through the nose.
4 Repeat rapidly for three cycles of around 20 breaths.

The benefits of breathing exercises

Practising any of these exercises regularly will help you to re-train your breathing and will also give you positive techniques to deal with stress and anxiety. Each of the exercises should also increase your overall energy levels. To gain maximum benefit from them, attend a yoga class initially, as this will help you to learn the different breathing techniques properly with someone on hand to guide you. You can then continue using them at home.

More on pranayama

Yogic breathing takes into account which nostril we are breathing through most at any one moment. The same sort of rules apply to our breathing patterns as to our left and right brain functions (see pages 24–5). The right side represents the moon – calm, intuition, emotion, and relaxation. The left represents the sun and the hot, masculine, aggressive side.

Apparently, whether we breathe predominantly through the right or left nostril changes naturally all the time, but if one becomes over-dominant it can cause problems. For example, breathing too much through the left nostril can make us vulnerable to fatigue and depression. When doing the exercises, try to concentrate on breathing through both nostrils as evenly as possible.

Do you find it hard to be calm?

Do you have trouble concentrating your mind?

Do your joints feel stiff all the time?

Yoga

Yoga is a system that was devised in India thousands of years ago for healing and rejuvenating the mind, body, and soul. It can offer support on all these levels, through meditation, exercise, and breathing, and so is useful whether we are in a low mood or not. But if the integrated philosophy seems too esoteric for you, start with a class that teaches basic yogic poses, which help free our body energy and promote overall calm.

How it works

Yogic *asanas* are said to work on balancing the subtle energy system of the body, which is made up of *chakras* and *nadis*. There are seven *chakras*, or energy centres, which run through the body from bottom to top: base, sacral, solar plexus, heart, throat, brow, and, the highest one, the crown chakra (see box on page 125). These chakras are linked by *nadis*, the energy channels that send *prana*, the body's vital energy, round the body (there are said to be 72,000 of these). The *nadis* correspond to the acupuncture meridians in the body.

Types of yoga

There are many different forms of yoga, which all draw on one another. Yogi Patanjali was the first to define eight steps for achieving spiritual enlightenment in his *Raja Yoga Sutras*. This 5000-year-old text includes principles such as truth, non-violence, cleanliness, a healthy body, study, and concentration of the mind. *Raja* yoga follows a psychological approach to learning how to control the mind.

In the West the most commonly practised form of yoga is *Hatha* yoga, which is a form of *Raja* yoga, but has its emphasis on balancing the physical body. The twisting, bending, and stretching exercises, or *asanas*, if practised regularly, are said to improve the function of the glands and regulate hormone production, as well as promote joint flexibility, particularly in the spine, and muscle strength. The movements within this form of yoga are slow and relaxed, and mainly deal with breathing and mental concentration.

Asanas There are 12 basic *asanas*, which means "steady pose" in Sanskrit, but there are many variations to each that can be learned gradually as we develop our flexibility. Although they appear to be working primarily on the physical body, regularly performing a programme of *asanas* gives benefit along the same lines as shiatsu massage and acupuncture, freeing up the body's *prana*, balancing emotions, and improving the overall oxygen flow round the body.

Kundalini This is our spiritual energy potential, and the yogis say that it lies dormant in the base chakra at the bottom of the spine like a coiled serpent. But practising yoga can awaken this spiritual energy, and it then rises up through the seven chakras, to stimulate higher states of consciousness.

Calming the mind

Stress is a normal part of life, but how we deal with it can be the difference between functioning well and falling into a depressive state. One of the problems is that our minds are always racing, and are constantly being bombarded by noise and information. Actually taking an hour once or twice a week to learn how to calm our minds can have a lifelong benefit, especially now that we live in such a busy world.

Because the yogic system of exercise is part of a deeper spiritual tradition, which believes that our physical body is the temple for our spirit, there is great emphasis on combining bodily movements with deep breathing techniques. Concentrating on the steady flow of breath in and out of our body as we practise *asanas* is a form of meditation, intended by the yogis to help us on the path to spiritual enlightenment. But it also has the benefit, even at a beginner's level, of soothing the distractions that clutter our mind and make us tense.

Learning how to do yoga

Yoga is not merely a set of exercises, like a sequence of aerobics is. Because it is an integrated mind, body, and spirit system, it is best to start practising yoga with a teacher who can explain the fundamentals of exercise and breathing properly. This can be done individually, or in a class. Such classes are not competitive in any way, and you are free to work at your own pace. After you have mastered the basic techniques, you can then practise yoga on your own if you prefer. The beauty of yoga is that you can take it to any level that you like, and can also continue to reap the benefits well into old age.

Evidence

A study published in the *British Medical Journal* had been carried out in 1985 in an attempt to discover the health benefits of yoga. The study involved 53 men and women who suffered from bronchial asthma and a separate control group with a similar severity of the illness. The people in the control group were given only drugs, while those in the other group took the drugs but also had two weeks of yoga meditation, exercise, and devotional sessions. They were asked to do yoga for 65 minutes a day. The results of the study showed that those who performed yoga as well as taking medication had fewer asthma attacks and needed less drug treatment afterwards than the control group did.

Energizing pose

This exercise is a very simple adaptation of the basic *asana*, "salutation to the sun". It increases lymphatic drainage and helps pump stagnant blood round the body so it is very good for depressive lethargy.

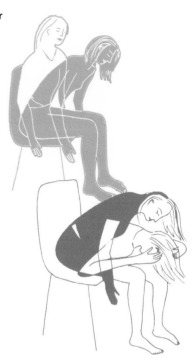

1 Sit comfortably on the edge of a chair with your knees apart and your feet firmly on the floor.

2 Sit up straight in the chair but relax your shoulders.

3 Tuck your chin in and gradually roll/move your body down between your knees, letting your arms hang loose towards the floor.

4 Now massage your scalp in firm circles with both hands as your head hangs down. This increases the blood flow and washes away any stagnation.

5 Drop your hands to hang loose again and stand up gradually, with your head still flopped forward and your knees slightly bent to take the pressure off the lower back.

6 Roll your spine up until you are standing straight.

7 Place your hands on your back, just below your waist, with your fingers pointing down, and bend backwards, stretching your shoulders wide, with your head back, and mouth and throat open.

8 Hold this position for a moment, then come back to a normal standing position.

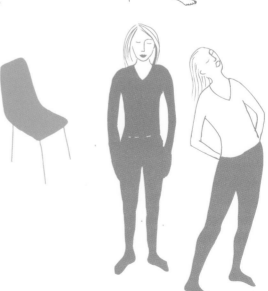

Relaxation

Yoga is not just about strength and flexibility, but also about relaxation. Again, this works on finding a balance. Too much exercise without the corresponding rest is as bad for us as doing no exercise at all, as our bodies have no opportunity to recharge their batteries. When we are depressed we often hold ourselves in a permanent state of tension, using our bodies as a protective barrier for our feelings. This can drain our energy and create all sorts of muscular pain and stiffness. We may then resort to alcohol and drugs to find the illusion of relaxation. Yoga is a better option. There are many simple poses that help relax the mind as well as the body. Try the ones shown here to begin the process. They are suitable for anyone.

Relaxation pose

This pose is specifically used to induce relaxation, and to allow the flow of *prana* round the body.

1 Lie flat on your back on the floor, with your legs straight and your feet at least 0.5m (2ft) apart.
2 Rest your arms by your sides, with your palms up at an angle of about 45° to your body. Try not to put any effort into the pose.
3 Now breathe as naturally as you can, focusing your mind on the rise and fall of your abdomen.
4 Stay like this for at least 10 minutes if you can.

Do the relaxation pose any time you are feeling stressed and tense and the energizing pose when you are feeling stuffy and lethargic or at the start of the day to get yourself moving. The more you do them the more you will feel the benefits.

The benefits of using these poses

If you are stiff and unused to exercise, these yoga poses can seem almost impossible and your yoga teacher can appear to be dauntingly supple. But yoga is a gradual strengthening and releasing process that can take years to master fully so don't be put off. The benefits, even at beginner level, will also be quickly apparent. It is important not to push your body to do more than it is ready for, and try to remember that you are not competing with anyone.

Do you lack self-confidence?

Do you find it hard to make decisions?

Do you feel out of balance?

Tai chi

Tai chi, which is also known as T'ai chi chuan and Taijiquan, is an excellent discipline for a person who is suffering from depression, because it increases the flow of energy, or "chi", around the body as well as promoting relaxation and calming the mind. Practised regularly it can build self-confidence and decisiveness, and it can also help sufferers to avoid depression in the future.

How it works

Through the practice of slow, fluid movement, correct posture, and breathing techniques, Tai chi increases the blood circulation to the brain and other internal organs, and promotes the flow of subtle energy, chi, round the meridians, or energy points, in the body. This improves the function of the immune system and, as a result, also protects the body from disease.

Tai chi also relieves stress by teaching us how to relax properly. The sequence of movements involved is designed so that the body flows in a single unit, likened to the flow of a river, but the lower half of the body is always firmly rooted in the earth.

Martial arts

Martial arts such as Tai chi were developed by the Taoist monks living in seclusion in the Wudang mountains of China many centuries ago. Although it is thought that the training evolved over many years, with input from various people, the man most credited with the creation of Tai chi is Chang San Feng. He combined the healing tradition of Chi kung with established movements and breathing techniques used by Taoist monks.

There are "internal", or soft, martial arts, and "external", or hard, ones. The internal ones include Tai chi and Chi kung, and the external ones include Kung Fu and Karate. Although both systems have the ultimate aim of improving and developing the strength of our mind, body, and spirit, they take slightly different routes to the same end. Soft styles work on our internal organs first, while hard styles begin by building external muscle strength.

What exactly is Tai chi?

"Tai chi" is the name of the circular Yin Yang symbol that has become popular as an emblem of the New Age movement and it represents the principle of balance in all things. The Chinese martial art of Tai chi stems from the ancient Chinese philosophy, Taoism. The most popular internal martial art in the world, Tai chi is practised extensively all over China, and is becoming very popular in the West. It is also called a moving meditation as it promotes clarity and calm in the same way that meditation does. It helps us to focus on improving our own inner awareness too.

Relaxing Tai chi generates the flow of energy in the torso with special breathing techniques, then sends the chi off to the limbs and the head by strong waist movements. During this fluid sequence of movement the body is relaxed and grounded, so that tension in the muscles does not impede the flow of chi. If our bodies are in a state of relaxation, then we are also able to relax our minds, and can allow tension and stress to be released.

How to practise Tai chi Books can tell us about the history, philosophy, and techniques of Tai chi, but it is not possible to master the art without instruction from a qualified teacher. There are many different forms of Tai chi, such as Yang, Wu, and Chen, and you should find the one that makes you feel the most comfortable. Unlike many forms of exercise, it is flexible and progressive and can be taken to any level you desire. This makes it ideal for everyone, especially if you are just starting to exercise and want to ease your muscles in gently.

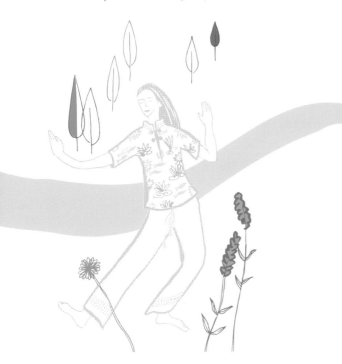

Evidence

An American trial in Atlanta Georgia in 1996 showed that the regular practising of Tai chi relaxed the muscles and the nervous system, which improved metabolism and enhanced the immune system.

Yin and Yang

The Chinese spiritual philosophy called Taoism, developed over thousands of years, believes that everything has its opposite, or balance. This is easily illustrated: life and death, male and female, night and day, and cold and heat to name a few examples. We can't have one thing without the other, and the flow of life is determined by the interchange and balance between the Yin and Yang in our bodies.

Illness is thought to come about when this balance is upset. A Yin condition occurs because there is not enough chi, or energy, in the body. A Yang condition is brought about because there is too much of this energy. Soft martial arts, such as Tai chi, can achieve and maintain this balance, so that they not only help to heal us when we are ill, but can also be a preventative measure to stop us getting ill in the first place.

Release your 'chi' with the soft, fluid movements of this internal martial art.

Are you anxious and stressed?

Do your energy levels feel low?

Do you feel apathetic?

Acupuncture

Acupuncture is one of the components in the ancient healing system, Traditional Chinese Medicine, known as TCM. Many of us in the West are unnecessarily squeamish about having needles inserted at the meridian points on our bodies, but the Chinese have successfully practised such techniques for thousands of years in order to balance the body's energy and relieve pain.

How it works

The balance of subtle energy, or chi, in our bodies is thought by TCM to be central to our health and happiness. Chi flows through our body along 12 invisible, paired channels, called meridians, each linked to a body organ. Along each meridian is an acupoint and there are up to 500 in all. Stimulation of these acupoints, either by the insertion of needles, or the application of pressure, heat, or an electrical charge, releases blocked chi and rebalances the body.

The principles of acupuncture

Taoism, which is central to Tai chi, is also the philosophy behind TCM and acupuncture. The balance of the complementary Yin and Yang in the body is what ensures the smooth flowing of chi (see box on page 83). Disruption, when either the Yin or Yang becomes dominant, can result in physical illness or emotional disorders, such as depression. Half of the meridians in the body represent Yin, including the heart, spleen, kidney, and liver. The other half represent Yang, and include the stomach, large and small intestine, and bladder. But the meridians are all interconnected, so a problem in the lung may, for instance, benefit from acupuncture on another meridian.

Acupuncture and depression Although the science behind the theory of meridians is not completely established, it is thought that acupuncture stimulates the release of chemical messengers, such as serotonin and noradrenaline, by its action on the nervous system. However, even though the technique is not fully understood, it has been shown to reduce anxiety and stress.

Electro-acupuncture This technique involves passing a small electrical current along the acupuncture needle, and has been indicated in Chinese studies as an effective treatment for depression. So far this is only an indication, not a proven theory.

Visiting an acupuncturist

A TCM practitioner will first make a diagnosis by taking your pulse and looking at your tongue, eyes, and skin. He or she will then insert very fine, stainless steel needles up to 2.5cm (1in) long into the acupoints that they feel are relevant to your condition. Between one and 16 needles can be used during a session, which will normally last for at least half an hour. The length of time the needles are in place varies too, from a few seconds to anything up to an hour.

Some people say it is a little painful or tingly when the acupuncture needle is first inserted, although others say that they don't even know it is happening. Reactions to a session also vary, although many people experience tiredness for a few hours after acupuncture. The number of sessions needed depends on many factors, including the severity of your problem and your general emotional and physical health, but expect to have at least 10 sessions. Before you embark on them, make sure that your practitioner is a fully qualified acupuncturist.

Acupressure

If the thought of needles makes you keel over with fright, it may be worth investigating acupressure. This therapy, which is thought to pre-date acupuncture, is also part of TCM and it addresses the same philosophy as acupuncture, but uses massage techniques instead of needles to release the flow of chi along the body meridians. It is said to be particularly effective in helping alleviate depression, although no one knows why.

Although this is a technique that can be self-administered, it is probably easier and more effective if done by a practitioner, especially if you are suffering from a complex illness like depression. The acupoint is usually quite tender when pressed, so it is not difficult to locate. Using fingers and thumbs, pressure is applied, then, maintaining the pressure, the point is massaged with quick, vigorous strokes. The length of time working on one point varies depending on what condition you have. Shen tao and shiatsu massages are both forms of acupressure (see pages 118–19), so you might consider consulting a therapist from one of these disciplines about your low mood state.

Five elements theory

Wood, fire, earth, metal, and water are the elements that form the TCM classification theory that is used in the diagnosis of disease. The organs of the body and the emotions and senses are all related to, and governed by, one of these five elements.

Each element therefore has a Yin organ and a Yang organ in the body with which it is linked, as well as specific emotions, tastes, and seasons. For instance, the earth element is represented by the following: the spleen is the Yin organ, the stomach is the Yang organ, and the emotion is worry. Earth's taste is sweet and the season is Indian summer.

All this has an effect on the type of treatment that is given and it therefore forms a diagnostic part of a traditional Chinese acupuncture session.

Evidence

A study recorded in 1986 in the *Journal of Traditional Chinese Medicine*, which was done in China and carried out on 142 car factory workers, found that daily acupressure kept up for 21 days resulted in improved sleep patterns for the majority of the group.

Do your muscles ache?

Do you have a stiff neck or shoulders?

Do you feel exhausted?

Physical relaxation

There is a big difference between healthy relaxation and exhaustion. We might think we are relaxed when we are slumped in front of the television, or even lying in bed, but often our bodies are scrunched and tense, and our brains are still whirring with stressful, unhappy thoughts. When we are depressed, although we feel lethargic and are unable to actually do anything, we are not necessarily relaxed.

How it works

Tension in the surface muscles of the body is a natural response to stress. When our muscles are tense we tend to take shallow breaths and, as a result, reduce the oxygen supply to our brain. Tense muscles promote stiffness and pain, which makes us even more tense. Focusing on how our body feels, consciously relaxing our muscles, and breathing deeply for short periods is a technique that, once mastered, can re-educate our bodies to deal with stress.

Recognizing tension

We often don't realize how tensely we hold ourselves. When we suffer from depression there can be a tendency to see our body as if it were a shell protecting us from the outside world. We also resort to repetitive movements, such as jiggling a knee, or dragging one foot back and forth under the desk. A very common movement is to clench our teeth. Take a moment to focus on your body and see if there are any obvious areas of tension, such as in your shoulders. Let them go heavy and loose, wriggle your body around into another position, and remember to check for tension again in half an hour. You will probably be surprised at the amount of tension that you carry about with you every day.

Progressive muscle relaxation

We must all take time out to re-energize our bodies, or we will begin to get tired and ill and won't be able to work effectively (see box, right). The first thing to do is to set some time aside for learning how to relax. It doesn't have to take more than 15 minutes a day, but it's better not to wait until you are in bed at night, unless you are suffering from insomnia, because you will probably fall asleep and the beneficial effects will be wasted. Rather, find a quiet spot some time during the day. This is obviously not always easy, but you will not relax properly with the television on, the children rushing round you vying for your attention, and the telephone ringing. Here is a simple technique to try during your relaxation time.

1 **Make the room warm and quiet. Lie on your back on the floor, and let your arms and legs flop away from your body.**
2 **Breathe slowly and deeply with as little effort as possible. Focusing on your breath (see pages 74–7) is a very useful way to calm your mind and begin the relaxation process.**
3 **Start the technique with your feet. Deliberately tense them to begin with and feel the tension – actually concentrate on holding your muscles stiff as you breathe in and out.**
4 **Then, on an out breath, let the tension go so that your feet flop. If it helps you to concentrate then say "relax" to yourself as you breathe out.**
5 **Now move up your body to focus on your calves, thighs, abdomen, chest, arms, hands, and neck, each in turn, to repeat the process of tensing and relaxing every muscle in your body, and then finish with your face. You can take as long as you like to do this exercise but ensure that you really concentrate on each group of muscles and specifically think about how they feel, both when they are tense and when they are floppy.**

You learn from this simple technique what your body feels like when it is really relaxed. The more you practise it, the more quickly you will recognize when you are getting tense. And, once mastered, you can use this technique anywhere: at the office, on the train, even when walking around – you don't have to lie down to do it. If you nip tension in the bud, the negative effects, such as muscle stiffness and trapped energy, will be minimized.

As we keep saying, our mind and body are inextricably linked. When we are depressed we hold onto negative thoughts. Negative thoughts promote physical tension, which in turn promotes exhaustion. To get out of this vicious circle we can focus on relaxation instead. Concentrating on our bodies and breathing, using the method described above, means letting go of negative thoughts. With practice, you will be able to deflect the spiral of negative thoughts before it takes hold of you.

Deep muscle relaxation

For a system of deep muscle relaxation combined with breathing and meditation, try Tai chi, yoga, or Aikido. These are all disciplines that can offer a complete re-education of the way that we treat our bodies.

Finding the time

It is easy to think that there is no time to relax, as there is just too much to get done. Many of us who experience low moods suffer from the being-busy-all-the-time syndrome. We have to prove how useful and efficient we are, because we don't really believe in ourselves. Relaxing can almost seem like a sin.

But long-term physical tension wears each one of us down, blocking the energy flow through our bodies and so reducing the amount of energy that is available for doing what we want, or need, to do. Therefore it is actually extremely important to make time to relax, so that we can be as effective as possible throughout the rest of the day.

Do you wake up much too early each morning?

Are you often irritable during the day?

Do you worry about not sleeping?

A good night's sleep

Sleep is the time when our body can regenerate itself. Lack of sleep makes us short-tempered, over-anxious, and vulnerable to ill health, and our work and relationships can suffer too. It is also a vicious circle; the less we sleep the more we worry about not sleeping, and the more we worry the less we sleep. Sleeplessness is a symptom of depression (particularly early waking) and it can be very debilitating and exhausting.

Circadian rhythm

Also known as our "body clock", our circadian rhythm is the 24-hour cycle linked to the rotation of the earth, which tells us when to sleep and when to wake. It is thought that the circadian rhythm of depressed people is out of synchronization. Although there is no proven cause or effect, the production of neurotransmitters and hormones that affect depression, such as serotonin and cortisol, is also closely linked to our circadian rhythm.

REM and non-REM sleep

Rapid eye movement (REM) is the state during which a person dreams whereas non-REM sleep is the time when the body has a chance to regenerate. Normally a person will fall into a deep non-REM state at the beginning of the night, followed by around four or five periods of REM states, which lengthen towards waking, but no one is sure how we benefit from these alternating states. Many, including Austrian psychoanalyst Carl Jung, believe that dreaming is a way of airing our subconscious; of looking over our emotional worries in a safe place.

Research has shown that depressed people have different patterns of REM sleep than others do. Depressed people appear to enter the REM state very early in their sleep cycle, depriving them of the regenerative non-REM sleep. Although both states are important, it is a disruption of the balance that causes problems and makes the sufferer feel exhausted and desperate.

Manipulating the sleep of a depressed person has been shown to have some success in improving sleep patterns, certainly in the short term. This involves depriving the person of sleep either partially, by letting them sleep for no more than six hours, or totally for a night at a time, until the sleep cycle readjusts. This is best done under careful supervision.

Insomnia

Some of us are light sleepers, while others sleep through absolutely anything. However, most of us have suffered at some stage from sleepless nights. Here are some of the reasons why:

Worry Most people can't sleep because they are worried about something. We either fail to fall asleep or wake in the night and can't get back to sleep for ages, only to fall into a deep sleep just before we have to get up. We are then groggy and tired.

Depression Depressed people often suffer from a very specific sleep pattern. They wake too early in the morning and can't get back to sleep. This can cause real distress.

Stimulants When we are worried or depressed, we often turn to caffeine and alcohol to get us through the day but too much of either interferes with our sleep as they are stimulants.

How much sleep do we need?

Everyone has different sleep requirements – some people are chirpy on five hours but others feel scratchy with less than ten. Eight hours seems about right for most of us, but it is the quality of sleep that matters most. A deep, uninterrupted sleep for six hours will leave us feeling better than 10 hours of tossing and turning with periods of wakefulness. A problem with sleeping is one of the first symptoms experienced by a depressed person.

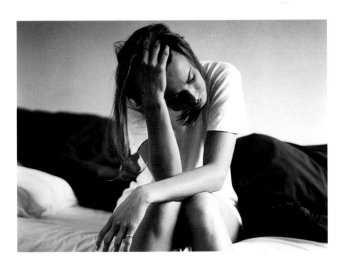

Tips for ensuring a good night's sleep

- Exercise each day.
- Wind down before bedtime with a warm bath and avoid any stimulating activity in the hour before you go to bed. Try to go to bed at roughly the same time every night and don't catnap in the afternoon.
- Avoid eating a large meal late at night and don't drink alcohol or caffeine. Have a warm, milky drink and a biscuit instead.
- Ventilation in the bedroom is important and so are suitable bedclothes for the time of year.
- Place a pad and pencil beside your bed. If you wake up and start worrying, write your worry down and decide to deal with it in the morning.
- Relax using the technique on page 87 in bed.
- Valerian, see page 63, is a herbal sleep remedy that provides a good quality of sleep without the "hangover effect" the next morning. Take an hour before bedtime. (This remedy usually takes up to two weeks to have an effect.)

If you have tried all the above and still can't sleep, ask your doctor for help. You may need to use conventional medication for a short while to set your sleep pattern straight again.

Lack of sleep can make you irritable and susceptible to illnesses, so finding time to relax and get a good night's sleep will improve your well-being.

Changing
your mind

Mind control summons up images of dubious cults, science fiction, and spy masters. Many of us believe that we have no control over the way we think and feel, although we accept that we control the way we behave. We acknowledge that we have a mind, a body, and a spirit, but in the West we don't relate one to another. So if we have depression, we take Prozac and hope the symptoms will go away. This is ignoring the example of the most enduring systems of medicine, such as Traditional Chinese Medicine, Ayurveda, and homeopathy, which firmly believe that all aspects of the ill person's life are relevant to the disease and look to treat the whole person.

Perhaps we are afraid that if we believe we have some control over our minds we will be blamed for being ill. But we are not to blame for being depressed, and can do much for ourselves by understanding why we are feeling so low. We can also perhaps learn ways in which we can prevent depression occurring again.

There are long-term strategies that can make us more familiar with the workings of our mind and offer ways to control our response to the stresses and strains of life. For example, we can calm our minds through meditation and visualization, understand what makes us stressed and develop ways to avoid or deal with it through hypnotherapy, and realize where our attitudes to ourselves and others come from to change the way we react through Cognitive Behavioural Therapy. These are just a handful of the helpful techniques and therapies discussed in this section.

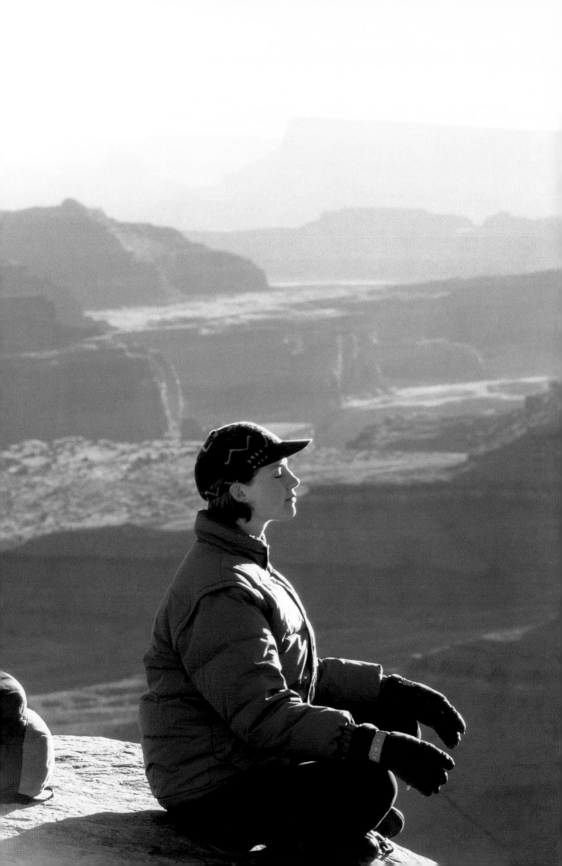

Is your mind cluttered with too many thoughts?

Can you deal with stress effectively?

Do you feel out of control?

Meditation

Meditation is extremely useful for those of us suffering from low mood states as it clears the mind of daily clutter to achieve a state of relaxed awareness. It can be immensely helpful as a technique for healing and de-stressing our mind and body, as well as being a tool for greater self-awareness. In the same way that we are what we eat, many would add that we are also what we think about.

How it works

There are four different patterns of brainwave. Beta waves, which occur during the normal waking, active state, are measured at around 20 Hertz (Hz). Alpha waves, which are associated with a quiet, meditative state, are measured at around 10Hz. Theta waves are produced during hypnosis, deep sleep, and meditation, and are found at around 4Hz. Delta waves, the lowest brainwave vibration, are found in the deepest states of meditation and sleep when a person has lost touch with outside reality. They are measured at under 4Hz.

When the brain goes into the alpha wave pattern during meditation, the mind becomes relaxed but stays alert, a state that allows the body to relax as well. In this place, the body's energies flow more freely.

Who meditates?

Most religions and philosophies practise meditation in one way or another. In the West we see it as an Eastern discipline tied up with yogis and gurus, but the prayers and chanting that are part of most church services are also forms of meditation.

Anyone can meditate; you don't have to believe in any particular philosophy. It offers a moment in the day when your mind can stop racing round, and provides a bit of peace and quiet instead. Meditation is a moment when you can control your mind instead of it controlling you. Regular periods of practising meditation produce clear thinking, greater energy, and the ability to deal with stress. Research also shows that it can be extremely effective in reducing anxiety and depression in most people (see box, right).

Mantras A mantra is a word or phrase that is used as a focus for meditation instead of an object. The most well known are probably the Hindu "OM" and "Hari Krishna", which is chanted by followers of the Krishna Consciousness Movement. You can use any word that means something special to you. The idea is to repeat the word or sound over and over until your mind gives up and becomes still. You can repeat the mantra silently, or out loud in a meditation group.

Koans These are meditation aids used by Zen Buddhists. They are riddles based on ancient Buddhist wisdom that cannot be answered except by deep self-realization. One example is "Who am I?"; only endless contemplation of such a question will provide the tranquillity of mind to understand the answer.

How to meditate

There are lots of classes and teachers to help you grasp the techniques of meditation, and a class or two to get you going is a good idea. But you could try starting with this simple meditation exercise. No special clothes or equipment are necessary.

1 Find a space where you won't be interrupted for 30 minutes.
2 Sit comfortably in a chair with your body well supported and relaxed, and your feet grounded on the floor while your hands are placed in your lap.
3 Breathe in and out through your nose, with your mouth closed. Try to make your breathing as effortless as possible.
4 Think of an image that you like, such as a rose or a tree.
5 Close your eyes and focus your mind on your chosen image as you breathe slowly in and out. In your mind's eye see its shape, colour, and experience how it feels and smells.
6 As you become distracted, which you will be, and your thoughts return to servicing the car or what to have for dinner, don't try to push these thoughts away. The more you try forcing them out, the longer they will linger. Acknowledge them as if they were performers filing across a stage. Watch them cross, say goodbye to them, and return to your image.
7 Stay as relaxed and still as possible for 10 minutes at first, breathing rhythmically and focusing on your image. After the first few times, sit for longer – 15–20 minutes is ideal.
8 When the time is up, take a couple of deep breaths and slowly open your eyes, giving yourself plenty of time to come back into consciousness. Stretch and then stand up slowly.

You will probably find it very difficult to do this exercise at first, and will be aware of how much your thoughts wander. But meditation is not about success or failure; it's about accepting what happens in our minds and beyond. If you persevere, you will find that you are better able to cope with stress as a result.

Evidence
Transcendental meditation, which was introduced to the West by the Indian yogi Maharishi Mahesh in the 1960s, has had over 500 studies done round the world that indicate its effectiveness, when practised regularly. These studies have shown that it increases self-actualization (emotional maturity, self-regard, and an adaptive response to challenges) as well as helping to reduce stress and anxiety.

One such study was done in America – it was carried out over three months and involved managers and employees of a manufacturing company. Those who regularly practised transcendental meditation throughout this time displayed increased relaxation and decreased anxiety and stress when compared to control subjects in similar jobs in the same company.

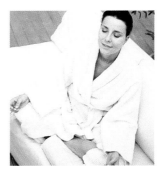

You don't have to be a guru to meditate. We can all find calmness and inner strength from the practice, however inexperienced we are.

Do you often have negative thoughts?

Do you find your life is confusing and painful?

Do you understand your dreams?

Visualization

Visualization can be a powerful technique for combating stress and for changing our negative attitudes. It is a form of meditation that uses our imagination to create a calmer, happier scenario than the one we are experiencing in real life. Repeated often enough, the body responds to the positive image rather than to the negative reality, and self-healing can occur.

How it works

No one quite knows exactly how it works, but it is thought that visualization acts on the right hemisphere of the brain, the side most associated with intuition and emotions. This, in turn, affects the hormonal and autonomic nervous system responsible for the functioning of the internal organs in the body – for example, changing the way we respond to stress.

Different uses for visualization

Visualization can be used to achieve many different ends, such as accessing healing power both for yourself and others, acquiring spiritual wisdom, or merely calming the mind.

Religious visualization Many different religions use forms of visualization. Tibetan Buddhist monks, for instance, visualize gods and goddesses to access their healing power, or to gain higher states of spirituality. Jewish mystics used visualization to

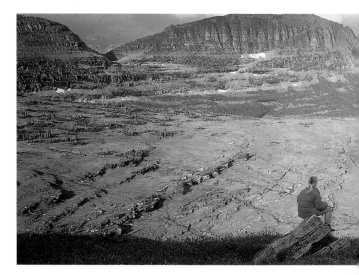

There are few things so uplifting to the spirits as a beautiful view, but when we don't have access to one it helps to be able to visualize it instead.

receive spiritual wisdom and psychic power from visions that came about through deepened levels of consciousness. Shamans, the spiritual healers common to Native American and Aboriginal tribes, regularly heal through visualization. In the West, a non-religious form of the technique is becoming increasingly popular.

Psychoneuroimmunology This refers to the process of using visualization to boost the immune system, which is also weakened when we are depressed. It has been particularly successful in treating cancer patients; a patient visualizes the destruction of the cancer cells, and the creation of more white blood cells to fight the invading tumour. Many cancer specialists worldwide include visualization as an important part of the treatment of the disease since it has been shown to aid healing.

When to use visualization
We can use visualization to help us in decision-making, stressful situations like job interviews and public speaking, or to generally improve our self-esteem. It is also helpful when we are depressed to use visualization to change the negative thought patterns we create about ourselves and the events in our lives. And, like meditation and breathing exercises, it encourages relaxation too. By being aware of the insights and messages our subconscious might evoke during the process of visualization, we can learn more about ourselves and the way we interact with others.

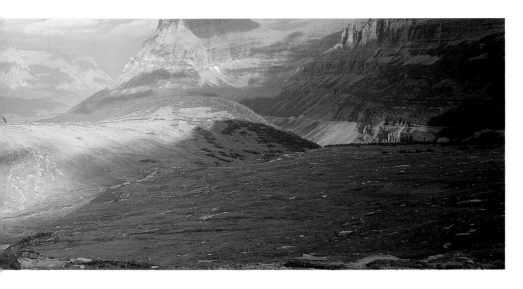

Visualization for stress relief You can either practise this technique with a therapist, who will guide you through appropriate visualizations, or can learn to do it yourself. Once you have mastered the technique you can use it any time if you are in a difficult situation or anticipate a problem.

1 Lie or sit in a warm, comfortable position, with your eyes closed. Make sure you won't be interrupted for 15 minutes.
2 Breathe deeply to help yourself relax and note if any area of your body is holding tension. If so, do the muscle relaxation on pages 86–7 before continuing.
3 Think of a beautiful, natural scene. It can be a real or imagined place such as a beach, a mountain scene, or a wooded glen. It may be somewhere that you have had happy times in the past. Above all it is a place where you are safe and is your own, unique, special place.
4 Now begin to feel what it is like to be there. Feel the warmth, the sunlight, the smell of the sea or wild flowers, and the tranquillity. How does the grass feel? Can you hear any birds? Feel the breeze on your cheek…
5 Breathe rhythmically, without effort, as you relax into the scene until you really believe you are there. If your mind wanders, bring it gently back to your special place.
6 When you are ready, bring yourself back to your current surroundings; take a few deep breaths and open your eyes.

Visualization for focused healing This particular visualization is for headaches or any other sort of physical pain.

1 Lie comfortably as before with your eyes closed.
2 Focus on the exact location of the pain and give it a colour and shape. For instance you could imagine it to be a red ball or orange spike.
3 Now imagine the object beginning to crumble and dissolve. See it gradually lose its shape and the colour fade.
4 When it is just a pile of dust, take a big, imaginary broom and sweep it out of your body until there is no trace of it left; imagine a gushing stream of water washing it away, or see the object turn into a liquid that drains out of your body.
5 Finally, imagine yourself without pain – healthy and happy.

With practice you will find that your mind is calm and your body relaxed after a visualization session. When you are under pressure, try to find time to do two sessions a day, one in the morning and one in the evening. It can be very helpful if you are suffering from insomnia too.

Dreams: unconscious visualizations

It is thought that dreams are an opportunity to gain insight into our subconscious and receive spiritual wisdom. In many cultures dreams are seen as divine guidance or cultivated as predictors of events. They are like unconscious visualizations.

When our sleep pattern is undisturbed we can expect to dream for up to five separate periods in one night. That's a lot of dreams in a lifetime, so the practice of interpreting our dreams makes sense. The wisdom that comes to us in our dreams comes from what Carl Jung called our "collective unconscious", the accumulation of aeons of spiritual knowledge. There are many different systems of dream symbolism, based on ancient spiritual traditions. The systems attach specific symbolism to the everyday objects we dream about – for instance, a baby symbolizes our innate creativity as it is the ultimate creation for human beings.

Another way to analyse our dreams is to ask ourselves how we felt and reacted in the dream. Were we overshadowed by those around us, unable to say and do what we wanted? Did we become angry when threatened? Our relationship to those around us in our dreams can be very telling. It's as if we have an opportunity to watch ourselves, and understanding our reactions can teach us a lot about our day-to-day behaviour. If the images, people, and places in your dream make no sense at all to you, then don't worry. If it's important you will dream it again, although it may be in a different form. It isn't a case of being right or wrong; you take from your dream what you can. Consult a dream analyst if you want specific help, or read one of the many books on the subject.

The more you practise these techniques, the more your mind will respond. Most people, at the very least, can benefit from the relaxation achieved from regular visualization sessions.

Remembering dreams

It is often difficult to recall a dream. The alarm goes off, the kids rush into the bedroom, and all is lost. The dream that seemed so vivid just a moment before is gone forever. We have less than a minute before it vanishes so it makes sense to have a pad and pen by the bed to write down your dream as soon as you wake up. The more you practise doing this, the easier it becomes to remember to do it as it will become part of your routine. You can also help yourself by saying before you go to sleep that you want to remember your dreams.

Do you suffer from long-term stress?

Do you bottle up your feelings?

Do you like to live on the edge?

Stress reduction

Stress gets a bad press these days, but there are times when it can be good for us. Being stimulated to achieve things often involves a degree of stress, and the adrenaline produced is what gets us through situations such as an interview or an exam. But if the stress is ongoing, the strain on the body can result in illnesses such as depression. However, there are things we can do to manage the amount of stress we experience.

How it works

The "fight or flight" response (see pages 26–7), which triggers the stress hormones adrenaline and cortisol, is vital for situations where we need short-term stimulation to cope with a challenge. But if these stress hormones continue to be produced over long periods, the body systems cannot cope and become impaired, increasing the likelihood of problems such as raised blood pressure, insomnia, anxiety, and depression. The immune system is also compromised, reducing antibody production and interfering with T-cell production (white blood cells), leaving the person vulnerable to disease. By using various techniques to reduce stress, we can stop the body from being stimulated to over produce the stress hormones.

Types of stress

There are major life stresses that all of us find it hard to cope with, such as bereavement. But these are usually short-term traumas, and, with the proper support, it is possible to deal with such stresses appropriately and eventually move on. The stress that needs managing the most is that brought on by the ongoing demands of everyday life.

Each of us finds different situations stressful, depending on our attitude to pressure and challenge. People who have a balanced, positive attitude to life can deal with much greater levels of stress than worriers and those with less confidence, who can view stress as an attack rather than a challenge.

We must also decide what value the stress in our lives has for us. Is it a subconscious desire for attention, because we need to feel needed, or have we become addicted to the excitement of living on the edge? If you are able to realize that you are stressed because being under such pressure suits you, then you can begin to address the reason for this as well as the stress itself.

Stress management starts with recognizing that we are stressed. This may seem obvious, but it is amazing how many of us are carrying around an unacceptable level of stress without being aware of it. We think we have adapted and may say things like "I'm used to working every weekend," but the damage to our body systems is nevertheless quietly accumulating.

Predisposing factors in stress

We've mentioned the fact that some stress is good for us, but what are the factors that can cause harmful stress?

Inability to switch off Some of us fill our days to bursting point. We are always on the run and never enjoy what we are doing as we're worrying about what we have to do next. Much of this type of stress is self-imposed. We identify too much with "doing" and not enough with just "being". It's almost as if we can't allow ourselves to have our own time. If you feel that this is describing you, ask yourself why you are always so rushed. Think about your day, and find something to delegate to someone else, even if it's only emptying the kitchen bin. And put aside an hour when you allow yourself to completely relax without feeling guilty about it.

Worry Nothing is gained by worry except more worry, stress, and insomnia. And often we can do nothing to change the situation we are in. If you can do something about it, then do it, and don't worry. If you can't, then there's not much point in worrying is there? But how do we stop? Try the suggestions over the page.

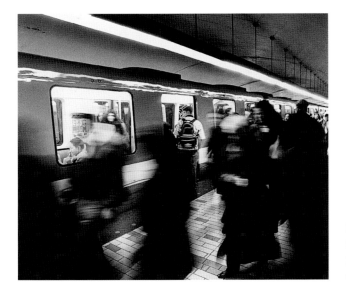

If we spend our lives rushing from place to place and never living in the moment, our health will begin to suffer.

STRESS REDUCTION

99

1 A time when many of us worry is in the middle of the night. For some reason the silence and the darkness magnify our problem, so we toss and turn. As soon as you start to worry, stop yourself with the promise that you will deal with it in the morning. Keep a pad and pencil by the bed if you like, and write the worry down so that you can deal with it the next day.

2 Don't take too much responsibility for other peoples' lives.

3 Don't allow a worry to build up into a monster. Face it, do what you can, and let the rest go.

4 Imagine the worst case scenario. For instance, you worry so much about being fired that it ruins your life. Could actually being fired be any worse? Would your world come to an end? Probably not.

5 Learn to talk about your worries to friends or relatives. The old adage "A worry shared is a worry halved" still stands good.

Situations out of our control, such as an unhappy marriage, not being able to find work, loneliness, and coping with a sick relative can add to our stress levels significantly. When the situation has gone on continuously for quite a while, we can find ourselves too worn out and exhausted to do anything constructive about it. The way to reduce this kind of stress-induced helplessness is to look at the small things we can do to improve the situation, instead of becoming stuck because we can't change the bigger ones. Make a list of the things about the situation that cause you the most unhappiness. For instance, if you are looking after a sick and elderly relative get a friend, or social services, to come in once a week so you don't have to miss the course that you really enjoy. Whatever stressful situation you find yourself in, it will make the burden seem lighter if you can just talk to someone. Have a good moan, and be brave enough to ask for support, both emotional and physical.

Suppressed anger Some of us tend to be reserved while others yell when the mood takes them and cry if they feel like it. The latter type deals with emotions much better than the first type. Keeping the lid on our emotions can be a great strain, and may result in inappropriate outbursts when we are under stress. Many of us also suffer from historically unexpressed anger generated in our childhoods, when we were too young to have a say in the way we were treated. This can surface as adults in a general raging at the world. Ask yourself these questions: when did you last lose your temper? Was it really justified? Do you lose your temper often? Do you think people are scared of your temper? Do you blame everybody but yourself when things go wrong? If you answer yes to these then you are either under a lot of stress or you have a deep-rooted problem with expressing your feelings, which may leave you vulnerable to stress in the future.

Strategies for coping with harmful stress

Once we have recognized that we are being subjected to harmful stress, there is a lot we can do to minimize the problem.

1 Decide what mileage, if any, you get out of the stress in your life. Does it provide attention or are you addicted to excitement?
2 Talk about your problems with a friend and ask for help.
3 Say no to things you don't need to do. Sometimes we get into the habit of thinking we're indispensable.
4 Don't bottle up your feelings. There's seldom a need to lose your temper if you deal with problems when they arise.
5 Be realistic about how long it takes you to get to places and complete tasks. Too much optimism in this area can cause stress.
6 Get into the habit of writing things down, such as phone numbers, appointments, shopping lists, and tasks for the day. Trying to remember things only adds to a stressful day.
7 If your work is the problem, seriously consider changing it, or ask if some of your workload can be delegated to others.
8 If your relationship is causing stress, talk about the problems with your partner and/or with a professional.
9 Make some time in the day when you are free to do what you want without feeling guilty. And make time to be with friends.
10 Eat healthily and regularly and avoid resorting to alcohol and stimulants to get you through the day.
11 Take time to wind down in the evening so that you have a better chance of a good night's sleep.
12 Develop a relaxation technique such as meditation or yoga.

Often just the recognition and acceptance of the fact that we are stressed can help to reduce its impact. It would be foolish to suggest that stress will miraculously disappear from our lives, but it is true that we can minimize it by the way that we deal with it.

Evidence

A New York study done in 1987 showed that students had lower antibody levels in their blood, which would make them more susceptible to infections, on the days when they felt stressed and depressed than they did on the days when they felt much more optimistic.

Are you addicted to something?

Are you generally an insecure person?

Do you panic in certain situations?

Hypnotherapy

Many of us are frightened by the thought of hypnosis as we worry that someone else will be in control of our minds. But hypnosis has been popular for centuries in some cultures and is used to help stimulate the body and mind to heal themselves. It has now also been adopted in the West for pain relief, helping with addictions such as smoking, reducing stress, raising self-esteem, and treating depression.

How it works

No one is quite sure how hypnosis works, but it seems to be effective on two levels. It induces a state of deep relaxation that promotes alpha waves, as in meditation (see page 92), which is, in itself, beneficial. And within this deep relaxation the conscious mind is circumnavigated, leaving the person open to suggestions that might change their unconscious attitude to their condition, which in turn may also affect their conscious perception.

In control

"You are getting sleepy", delivered with ponderous and sinister emphasis, has long been part of the comic tradition of describing hypnosis. But who is in control when we allow ourselves to be taken into a hypnotic state? Can we have our minds bent by unscrupulous practitioners to do and think things we would not otherwise want to?

The bond of trust between subject and therapist is key to the success of the technique. Hypnotherapists insist that not only is it impossible to hypnotize a subject unless he or she is willing to be hypnotized, but also that, once hypnotized, the unconscious mind will resist any suggestions that seem like unreasonable manipulation. However, it is essential to find a hypnotherapist who is qualified and reputable, because you need to trust them while they access your subconscious. If your therapist is using hypnotherapy for psychoanalytic purposes, for instance, and is taking you back to previous, buried traumas from your past, you may find the experience upsetting, and you need to know that you will be getting the proper level of support through this.

Although there is no scientific evidence that depression can be cured by hypnosis, the symptoms of low mood states, such as sleeplessness, anxiety, low self-esteem, and panic attacks, can be successfully modified with regular hypnotherapy. It is not, however, suitable for severe depression, psychosis, or epilepsy.

What happens during hypnotherapy

The therapist will make sure you are comfortable, either sitting or lying down. He or she will then take you into a level of trance through various suggestions, visualizations, and repetitions. You may not even be aware that you have entered the hypnotic state. It can feel a bit like the moment between waking and sleeping, when you are aware of the outside world, but are also disengaged from it. This induction can take a few minutes, or much longer, depending on your willingness to be hypnotized.

During the session, the therapist might get you to discover what it is that triggers your panic attacks, for instance, then will offer suggestions that change the way you view the trigger next time you are confronted with it. He or she might get you to associate a positive image instead of a negative one with the cause of your panic, to enhance your confidence in dealing with it.

There are various levels of trance induced during hypnosis, but they are ill defined, and there is debate about how many levels there really are. The more familiar you are with the process, the deeper you will be able to go, but the majority of treatments will be carried out in the medium levels of trance.

Many people going for their first hypnotherapy session are not aware at the time of treatment that anything significant has taken place, and only realize the effectiveness later on when they experience some improvement in their condition.

Learning the technique You can also learn how to hypnotize yourself. This can be particularly helpful for improving self-confidence, but it needs to be practised regularly before you will reap many benefits. The technique is similar to visualization and focused meditation (see pages 92–7). There are many tapes and books on the subject but you may prefer to consult a hypnotherapist for guidance. With a trained and respected practitioner to help them, many people find relief from anxiety, phobias, and depressive symptoms with this therapy.

Evidence
An Australian study done in 1978 used one session of hypnosis to treat 75 patients' smoking habits. This session involved ego-boosting and positive visualizations. Results showed that 45 patients stopped smoking straight away and, of these, 34 were still non-smokers six months later.

Mesmerism
The 18th-century Austrian doctor Franz Anton Mesmer first developed hypnosis in the West. His trance-inducing technique using magnets, known as "mesmerism", was immediately dismissed by many as being the work of a charlatan.

Do you have difficulty in thinking positively?

Do you suffer from a phobia?

Do you have trouble communicating with others?

Neuro-linguistic programming

Neuro-linguistic programming (NLP) seeks to change the way we view our lives by challenging the blueprint set up by our experiences. It teaches us to take control of our thoughts and emotions and is useful in treating many illnesses and emotional problems.

How it works

NLP is based around the premise that when we are faced with illness, either mental or physical, we often lose hope, and if we do this then our bodies also lose the ability to heal themselves. NLP sets out to give us the hope that nothing, including illness, is written in stone. It does this by promoting the idea that we can change our attitude and self-image to make life work for us, ie healthy patterns of behaviour and thinking bring about healthy physical and emotional effects.

Studying experience

John Grinder and Richard Bandler set out in the 1970s to study why successful people were so successful, and went on to work at the possibility of duplicating such people's technique for others to use. They based NLP on the study of how these effective people communicated using their bodies – eye movements etc – believing that these outward behavioural signs reflected each person's subconscious perceptions. These perceptions, good or bad, are, they believe, a self-fulfilling prophecy.

Representational systems

We use a combination of our five senses – visual, auditory, kinaesthetic (touch and internal feelings), gustatory (taste), and olfactory (smells) – to perceive the world. According to NLP, we all use these systems differently to create our own map of reality. So the same signal can be interpreted in many ways, based on our own experiences, opinions, and biases. How our map is built affects the way that we relate to the people and events in our lives, and also directs the results we obtain from the encounters. NLP believes that we can change that map until we get the result that we want. The varied techniques of NLP, such as word association (anchoring) and watching how a person moves their eyes (eye accessing cues), are used at a therapist's discretion. In order to explain how they work, we have chosen to discuss one of them in detail – "disassociating a situation". We tend to see what happens to us from the first-person perspective. If you re-experience a situation from the other person's point of view, it becomes disassociated and therefore open to change. For instance, imagine you have had a row with your mother. She is angry with you for being late for Sunday lunch. Take a few minutes to run over the row in your mind.

First re-experience it from your point of view, remembering how your mother reacted, looked, and sounded. Then change your position, and re-experience it as you think your mother might have, based on what you know about her. Ponder how you think she saw you, what she thought you were thinking etc. Lastly, clear that image and imagine what an outsider might have experienced watching you two row about your lateness. When you have all three images in your head, you will be able to be much more objective about how you and your mother were feeling. These different perspectives offer you the chance to understand yourself and others and make changes to your behaviour so that the next time you deal with the same situation you will be more effective.

Visiting an NLP therapist

A neuro-linguistic therapist will watch you closely as you describe your problems, and will analyse how you speak, how you hold your body, your facial expressions, and the words you choose. No assumptions are made about your communication, and the therapist will go on asking probing questions until she or he understands what is behind what you are saying. The therapist will then help you to remodel your attitudes and perceptions, replacing the negative patterns with positive ones, to bring about healing, change, and growth.

Many of the techniques of NLP are being used increasingly to improve communication skills in business, as well as personal, relationships. Since many of the problems we encounter are based in poor communication and understanding of others, you might find this therapy worth investigating for these benefits alone, although it will also help you to cultivate a healthier, positive outlook about yourself and others.

Presuppositions

Also known as "givens", presuppositions support the theory that change is both a possible and inevitable part of finding solutions to our problems. Here are some of the presuppositions used in NLP:

- Communication is more than what you are saying; it also involves body language.
- No one is wrong or dysfunctional. We all work perfectly to achieve what we are trying to achieve, even if this is destructive to our lives.
- We all have all the resources we need; we just haven't got them lined up right.
- The meaning of communication is the response you get.
- If you aren't getting the response that you want, then try something different.
- There's no such thing as failure, only feedback.
- Flexibility is the key to change.
- Every type of behaviour is useful in some context.
- If someone can do something, anyone can learn how to do it.
- Whatever we say or do, we all communicate.

Do you expect to fail when you try something new?

Do you believe that you can be happy?

Do you have friends who will listen to you?

Affirmations

It is easy to get into the habit of viewing the world with a negative mind set. Many of us do it without being aware that we are. And if we give out a negative message, we often get a negative response. This is disheartening both for us and for those around us. We can't force ourselves to be relentlessly jolly, but we can change the way we approach things, and will make our lives a great deal happier and healthier as a result.

How it works

It is very simple – if we are continuously negative, then the world seems to be a negative place and often the people around us react to us in the same negative way. By changing the way we approach life, from always being negative to being much more positive, we can actually change the outcome too. There has also been research that links happiness and positivity to the body's ability to heal itself.

Eastern philosophies

The East is ahead of the game when it comes to philosophies that promote positivity. What they all basically suggest is that we can take control of our lives to change them for the better.

Vedanta is a school of Indian philosophy. The writings that form this philosophy are found in the *Upanishads*, a collection of ancient spiritual teachings, and those who live by the tenets of Vedanta believe in positive thinking. They say that the fundamental problem we all face is that we usually feel inadequate. But our misguided solution, which we think will make us adequate, is to seek security (*artha*) and pleasure (*kama*). But they believe we can only become truly happy and free when we realize that no amount of pleasure or security achieves the goal of happiness. This liberation (*moksa*) comes about through meditation and teaching on our true nature.

Vipassana is a Tibetan Buddhist technique that uses affirmations to change the way we think. Most of us constantly sow the seeds of failure and low self-esteem into our lives. Faced with a challenge, many of us immediately tell ourselves we won't be able to do it. This is not helpful. If we think we will fail, then we will. According to the theory of Vipassana it is as simple as that. It's a case of we are what we think.

Using affirmations

If we make positive affirmations about the qualities that we would like to possess they will become a reality. So instead of thinking, "I'm hopeless with relationships", affirm to yourself "I am loving and worthy of love". Now this may sound phoney – how can you say something to yourself that you don't believe is true? Well, according to the Buddhist teaching, it is true, but you just haven't realized it yet. You are loving and worthy of love, but you have mislaid these qualities because the messages you have received about yourself have been negative ones.

Affirmations are very powerful, so it's important to be realistic in what you ask for because you just might get it. Write a list of all the qualities that you are seeking; such as confidence, popularity, money sense, and trustworthiness. This shouldn't be viewed as a wish list; it is a list to bring your hidden qualities to life. So begin your list with the words "I am...". For example, "I am a confident, popular person who is capable of trust and can earn enough money to stop worrying about the bills. This is what I deserve. May I be well and happy". Take your time while writing and, when you are happy with your affirmation, repeat it until you have memorized it. The more often you use it, the more successful the outcome will be. You can say it to yourself, or out loud, absolutely anywhere but make sure you repeat it in groups of seven. According to British Vipassana teacher Michael Kewley, this allows enough time for the positive energy of your statement to build and be more effective. At first you might hear a little voice telling you that your affirmations are not true. Ignore it and press on. It usually takes at least a month before you can expect to see a result but when aspects of your affirmation are well established, you can change them for others.

Learning from experience It is a great deal easier to be negative when you are on your own. How often have you felt overwhelmed with gloomy thoughts, then spoken to a friend who has put a different perspective on your problem and made you feel better? Whether alone or with friends, listen to how you interpret the events of your day, see how much of the negativity is justified, and then try to approach tomorrow with a more positive outlook, learning from the day that has just passed.

Evidence

A study done at America's Harvard University over a 25-year period, which was published in 1988, showed that male students who were pessimistic in outlook were more prone to ill health in later life than those who had an optimistic view of life.

"We are what we think. All that we are arises with our thoughts. And with our thoughts we make our world."
Sidhattha Gotoma,
The Buddha

Do you find it hard to accept a compliment?

Do you feel that the world is against you?

Do you always jump to negative conclusions?

Cognitive Behavioural Therapy

Cognitive Behavioural Therapy (CBT) has been shown to be particularly successful in treating mild and moderate depression. It sets about to change the negative way we often view our lives so that we can gain a more positive and healthy outlook.

How it works

The cognitive theory states that we can understand and control the negative thought patterns that were developed in our early childhood. These affect our emotions and behaviour so this therapy teaches techniques that offer more realistic ways to approach our lives. It uses a person's everyday experiences to highlight the problem and effect change.

Psychoanalysis versus cognitive therapy

Psychoanalytic theory believes that the root of all our neuroses lies in the hidden traumas of childhood. We cannot become aware of these traumas unless they are brought to our conscious mind through psychoanalysis, so we have no control over the negative thought patterns these traumas engendered. A psychoanalyst will therefore delve into the meaning behind the person's thoughts, rather than the thoughts themselves.

In the 1970s psychoanalyst Aaron Beck decided that this approach was wrong, and that the way a person thinks (not the hidden meaning) is the key to how he or she feels. He decided that we are, in fact, able to be made aware of how we are thinking and how that affects our life, and can then change it into something more realistic.

Beck's techniques have since been combined with the work of earlier behaviour therapists, who believed that behaviour is a learned response to past experience, and that it can be unlearned without delving into the past to discover why the original problem surfaced. The combined theories and techniques have evolved into Cognitive Behavioural Therapy. CBT does seem to be a more straightforward approach than psychoanalysis, and is also more easily grasped by the person engaging in the therapy.

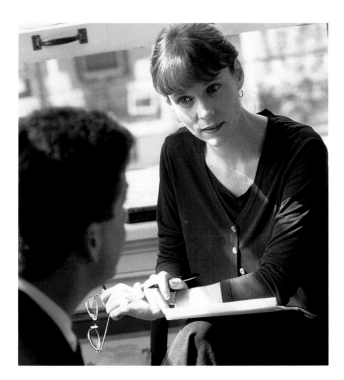

We can be encouraged to adopt a more realistic thought process by seeing a CBT therapist.

Some of the reasons for this include the following:

1 It is goal directed, offering techniques that involve adapting responses to the symptoms the person has presented with.
2 The sessions are structured, which often makes the patient feel more comfortable.
3 It is usually short-term; 10–20 50-minute sessions on average.
4 The patient contributes to the therapy by working in partnership with the therapist to bring about recovery.
5 Some studies that suggest that although CBT is slower in dealing with depression than taking an antidepressant drug is, it is more effective in preventing a later recurrence of the condition. However, CBT and antidepressant drugs do work well together, so a combination of the two may be effective.

The cognitive triad This three-pronged model was developed by Beck to describe the way a depressed person sees the world.

1 The depressed person tends to believe that what he sees as unpleasant experiences are the result of his own inadequacy.

The cognitive model of depression
Early experience leads to **dysfunctional assumptions**, which lead to **critical incident**. This then becomes **assumptions activated**, which turn into **negative automatic thoughts** that lead to **symptoms**.

So, for instance, Julie had a childhood where she was always being told she was stupid, not pretty enough, and clumsy. She assumes this to be true because it was her reality as a child. She then finds out her husband is having an affair. Her assumptions about herself surface: "Of course he is having an affair," she thinks, "because I am so ugly, stupid, and unlovable". She then spirals into a negative thought pattern about her own inadequacies and becomes depressed, sleepless, and physically ill.

"The way we think in turn affects our emotions and thus our behaviour."
Aaron Beck

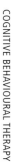

How do you think?

We are often completely unaware that we are thinking in a distorted way as we have probably been practising the same automatic, negative way of thinking unconsciously for years. Pondering a recent incident in your life, when you felt bad and unhappy with the outcome, can help you to discover your automatic thought patterns. Ask yourself the following questions:

- Can I see any evidence for the negative thoughts I have about this situation?
- Am I selecting this single incident and giving it a global significance it doesn't deserve, to prove how useless I am?
- Do I benefit in any way by holding onto these thoughts?
- Is it really all my fault?
- Could that person have reacted badly to me simply because they are having a bad day?
- Am I judging this situation based on all the evidence?
- If I do something badly, does it mean I do everything badly?
- Can I learn useful things from this situation?
- Am I ignoring the good things in my life?

2 The person believes that the world is against him, and is full of unattainable goals that make him feel a failure.

3 The future looks particularly bleak to a depressed person. He is unable to see how things might be better in the future, so he often sees no point in going on.

Distortions in reasoning

There are certain common types of mistake in reasoning that a person suffering from a low mood state makes when faced with everyday situations. These create unrealistic automatic thoughts, which in turn create gloom. Some of these are:

Jumping to conclusions This is when a person takes a small incident, or selects a fragment of an exchange, and infers a negative conclusion, even when there is no concrete evidence for this conclusion. *Example: Mary's boyfriend says he will call on Saturday, but he doesn't. Mary, who is already in a low mood, immediately decides that this proves he doesn't love her anymore and that no one else ever will. In fact, her boyfriend got drunk with a friend and forgot about his promise. Not great behaviour, but nothing to do with his feelings for Mary.*

Exaggeration This is when the depressed person blows a minor setback up into a major one, and is unable to evaluate the real significance of the event. *Example: John takes his driving test for the first time. He fails, and decides that there is no point in taking it ever again because he is a hopeless driver and will always fail it, despite the known fact that most people fail the first time.*

Never believing a compliment When we are depressed it is often difficult to accept the good things that people say to us. *Example: Sebastian's boss calls him in to tell him how well he handled their new clients. Sebastian, instead of believing the compliment, dismisses the praise and says to his work colleagues, "She probably just wanted to butter me up because she's not going to give me a raise".*

A cognitive therapist would help each of these people to recognize their patterns of mistaken reasoning and modify them, as well as to understand that the thoughts resulting from this mistaken reasoning are unrealistic and therefore unhelpful.

Going to a therapist

Seeing a therapist can feel very frightening. The thought of taking the lid off our pain can seem too difficult or even dangerous and we may ask ourselves the following questions. Will the therapist be able to cope? Will she think I'm a horrible and shameful person? If I get angry will I hurt her? These thoughts are normal, and the therapist will expect you to feel this way. It can be a tremendous relief to unload your fears to someone who accepts and understands the way you feel.

You might be asked to keep a diary of the week between the sessions you attend. This would include detailing times when you felt unhappy and couldn't cope, and other times when you felt better about yourself. Then the therapist may take one of the incidents and ask you how you felt, what thoughts you had, what those thoughts meant to you, and how you reacted. By doing this you will eventually be able to identify what triggers your bad feelings, and understand why they cause such feelings. The therapist might even draw a diagram to show you clearly how your thoughts and behaviour trigger each other in a predictable pattern. Using visualization, role play, and by examining the evidence and helping you generate alternative reactions, the therapist will aid you in changing and rectifying the distorted thinking that makes you vulnerable to your low mood states.

If you do not feel trusting and comfortable with the therapist that you initially choose, then find someone else. It is your prerogative to decide who you want to work with – just because you try a therapist once does not mean you should feel guilty if you don't think they are the person that you want to work through your problems with.

If you are suffering from mild or moderate depression, it is well worth considering Cognitive Behavioural Therapy, not only for the short-term treatment of your problem, but also to help you find strategies for coping with your life in the future.

Evidence

A Dutch study in 1995 took 79 people between the ages of 18 and 64 who had unexplained physical symptoms but scored high on the anxiety and depression scale. 39 of these people were given CBT. At the end of a six-month trial, the ones who had received the therapy had a higher recovery rate, less frequent symptoms, fewer social limitations, and less sleep impairment than the group that hadn't been given any treatment.

Sense
your mind

There are some nations that just aren't "touchy-feely". Others, however, throw their arms around each other in a greeting. If we are not used to much physical interaction we can become very isolated, as there is no one to give us an all-important hug.

We do all need some level of physical contact – it is a vital part of human interaction, and the physical approaches to healing such as massage, aromatherapy, and reflexology have long been recognized as having a deep effect on our emotional and spiritual health. They release tension and negative energy, stimulate the circulation, and encourage lymphatic drainage (this is the method that the body uses to get rid of toxins). The way that we respond to human touch during massage can also trigger the rush of mood-enhancing endorphins that lift our spirits.

Our eyes and ears are also important vehicles for relaxation and healing. Sufferers of Seasonal Affective Disorder (SAD) have been shown to benefit greatly from light therapy, and our minds do actually respond to colour and music far more than most of us are aware of. The success of music therapy is just one example of this.

Bombarded as we are by the noise and visuals of modern living, perhaps it is time to allow the sensual side of our nature to have more of an airing. Take time to smell the flowers, listen to some beautiful music, be more aware of the beauty around you, and feel the touch of someone you care for. Wake up your senses and give them a chance to make you feel better.

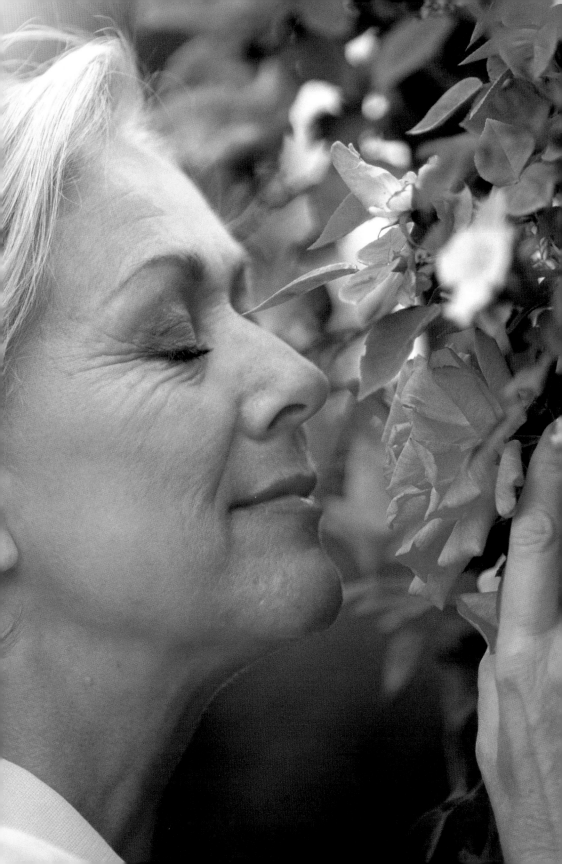

Are your spirits consistently low?

Do you find it hard to make decisions?

Do you feel that you haven't got any energy?

Aromatherapy

The essence of plants has been used for centuries in every culture – incense and perfumes are just two examples. Aromatherapy uses plant essences in a holistic approach to healing; seeking to balance the mind/body energies through baths, massage, vaporization, skin compresses, and ointments. Depression is seen as a state of imbalance and can benefit from the gentle application of essential oils.

How it works

Aromatherapy works on two levels. The massage technique employed is the touch element and this has been shown, in recent research using PET scans (see pages 24–5), to stimulate the brain. (This research was done in 1998 at the Institute of Neurology, London, England.)

Aromatherapy is also said to help rebalance the autonomic nervous system (responsible for involuntary, automatic activities such as the heartbeat, breathing, and digestion), which is upset during any illness.

Aromatherapy also delivers the healing properties of each plant's essential oils through inhalation and absorption into the skin.

Sense of smell

Humans are very sensitive to smells. Each one of us produces our own individual scent, known as a pheromone, and we can like or dislike someone, or even find them sexually attractive, because of their particular odour. A strong part of the bonding process between a mother and her baby is through their sense of smell. Any woman who has had a baby will remember how absolutely delicious their own baby smelled. Our sense of smell also protects us from danger by detecting smoke, gas, or food that has gone off. It can also be the most potent reminder of the past, evoking either pleasant or unpleasant memories.

It has been scientifically proven that smells create a profound psychological and physiological response. A scent stimulates the olfactory system in our brain, which then affects the limbic system (which is responsible for memory, emotion, and learning; see page 25). Endorphins are also triggered by scents, either to calm the brain or to increase activity.

Extracting and using essential oils

The concentrated oils extracted from plants can be found in various different parts. Depending on the type of plant, it may be the root, leaves, flowers, seeds, fruit, or bark that hold the oil. Generally, the oil is obtained through steam distillation,

Lavender

Some oils have multiple uses. Lavender was the oil that first alerted René-Maurice Gattefosse, the originator of modern aromatherapy, to the healing technique: he had burned his hand in a laboratory experiment and for some reason decided to plunge his hand into a vat of lavender oil. He discovered his burn healed remarkably quickly and well.

Lavender is an antiseptic, analgesic, and antibiotic, and it also relieves muscle pain, menstrual pain, child colic, and depression. Take a lavender bath before you go to sleep at night or put a few drops on your pillow and you will sleep much more soundly.

during which the plant is steamed and the resulting steam, which contains the essential oil, is cooled and then the oil is separated out. This is then usually mixed with a carrier oil, such as almond or sunflower, before use as it would be too potent on its own.

Absorbing the oils Aromatherapy oils are absorbed through inhalation during massage, through a vaporizer, in a scented bath, or from a pillow or handkerchief with a few drops on it.

Oils can also reach the internal organs and centres in the brain through the skin. Just as we sweat waste products through the pores in our skin, so we are able to absorb substances through them into our bloodstream. Skin patches, which are used for delivering hormones and anti-smoking and anti-alcohol drugs, use this method.

Visiting an aromatherapist

An aromatherapist will select the oil, or combination of oils, that are tailored to meet your individual needs. The therapist will not only be treating the symptom, but will enquire into your general emotional and physical health to determine the best scents to use. Sometimes a therapist will allow you to sniff a few scents to select the one(s) that feels right for you. As well as giving you massage treatment, he or she might suggest using the relevant oils in your bath or on your pillow at night. You should feel the beneficial effects of aromatherapy immediately, but for a longer lasting improvement, it is best to have regular weekly sessions until your body has achieved a more balanced state.

Aromatherapy for depression

Because low mood states have many different causes and manifest themselves in many diverse symptoms, from lethargy to anxiety, there is a wide range of essential oils available for alleviating and treating symptoms.
Camomile, **lavender**, and **sandalwood** each have antidepressant and sedative qualities within them.
Rose and **geranium** can help lift your spirits but do not have a sedative effect.
Jasmine is said to imbue confidence in dealing with difficult problems and can also help with self-esteem.
Neroli is excellent for alleviating the anxiety associated with depression.

Evidence

Trials done at the Middlesex Hospital in London, England in 1994, using cardiac patients, indicated that those massaged with neroli essential oil diluted in vegetable oil felt much calmer than those massaged with vegetable oil alone.

Are you happier in spring and summer?

Are you sluggish and overweight in the winter months?

Do you have difficulty waking in the winter?

Light therapy

Sunlight puts a spring in our step and lifts our spirits. The long hours of darkness in the winter months can create a desire to hibernate, but for those suffering from the depression known as Seasonal Affective Disorder (SAD), these short days have a much more devastating effect. One of the most effective treatments for this condition is daily exposure to filtered full-spectrum light, the closest thing to natural sunlight.

How it works
Bright white light, or full-spectrum ultra-violet filtered light, is almost the same as natural daylight, but it has had the potentially damaging ultra-violet rays filtered out. It is delivered to a SAD sufferer via lamps or a light box as a replacement for the daylight they require to balance their hormone production and stop them becoming depressed.

Evidence
According to studies from the University of Tulsa, USA, women whose choice of exercise exposed them to a relatively large amount of sun reported less depression in winter than women who exercised primarily indoors did.

SAD explained
Light enters the eye and stimulates the pineal gland, which controls the production of several brain chemicals. Serotonin, which is the "feel good" neurotransmitter implicated in raising our spirits, is produced more in the spring and summer along with the increase in hours of sunlight. Melatonin, also known as the sleep hormone because the pineal gland begins to secrete it during hours of darkness, has the opposite effect to serotonin, as it makes us feel drowsy and sluggish. When the balance of these two hormones is affected due to a disruption in sleep patterns or lack of light during short winter days, some of us become vulnerable to depression.

SAD has many of the symptoms of other forms of depression, such as lethargy, carbohydrate craving, fatigue, low moods, and difficulty in waking, but the sufferer noticeably improves when the days become longer in spring, and then goes into a downward depressive spiral again in winter. These seasonal and predictable cycles are what distinguish a SAD sufferer from a person with another form of depression.

Light deprivation
We are all vulnerable to light deprivation. Research has found that most of us spend 23 out of 24 hours indoors. Add to that

the fact that days are frequently overcast and short in winter and it is easy to understand why some of us can become depressed.

We measure light in a unit called a lux. The light at twilight measures just below 750 lux, while an indoor home is lit between 200 and 500 lux. A more brightly lit office is normally 400–700 lux. Obviously daylight varies depending on the weather and the time of year, but a spring day at noon could measure as much as 81,000 lux, and even at 5.30 in the evening it could still be 10,000 lux. So it is very important to get as much daylight as we can. Go out for a walk at lunchtime and walk home if you can.

Visiting a therapist

When visiting a light therapist, you will be positioned under lights, fully clothed, with your eyes open, for periods of time between 20 minutes and two hours. It is best to do this during the morning hours so that you are then brightened up for the rest of the day. The strength of the light and the time under it depends on the therapist's assessment of your condition, but a minimum of 2500 lux is required to have any noticeable effect. The therapist might also suggest you get a light box for home. You would need to sit in front of this for 20 minutes a day. The benefits are usually felt quickly, but the treatment has to be continued to maintain the improvement.

Using light therapy This therapy has other applications, such as using exposure to UV light to help in skin conditions like psoriasis, but American studies have shown UV-filtered broad spectrum light to be highly effective in treating SAD. Daily exposure is said to improve the condition in at least 85 per cent of people. The research done so far suggests that the ultra-violet component does not increase the antidepressant response to light therapy – it is the light itself that is important for this treatment. As UV has a toxic potential it is best avoided anyway, which is why the light used in light therapy is filtered first.

If you are prey to cyclical bouts of feeling low at the same time every year, light therapy should be able to help. You may have to use it regularly during the winter months for the foreseeable future, but the treatment will help to alleviate your symptoms.

Evidence
A study of 191 people with SAD, reported in the *Journal of Clinical Psychiatry* in 1999, showed that light therapy relieves suicidal ideation and produces clinical improvement in the majority of patients studied, and that the emergence of suicidal ideas was uncommon while they were treated with light therapy.

Coloured light therapy
Coloured lights have been shown to have beneficial effects on conditions such as anxiety and depression. Although it has long been observed that people respond in different ways to colour, coloured light therapy is a new development in the use of light therapy. Coloured strobe therapy shines different coloured flashing lights into the patient's eyes, and red light therapy has also been used to treat a variety of illnesses. Research and the practice of coloured light therapy is still, however, in its infancy.

Is your body often tense and stiff?

Do your muscles ache regularly?

Do you feel tired out all the time?

Massage

Massage is as much to do with the healing touch of the therapist as it is to do with muscle manipulation. Healing energy passes from the therapist to the client during a massage session, and the sensation of touch alone stimulates the systems of the body to aid in the healing process. Vigorous massage strokes also enable the muscles to be freed from stiffness and tension.

How it works

The skin is covered with thousands of nerve endings that convey the stimulation of touch through massage to all areas of the body. As a result, the flow of oxygen around the body is increased and the excretion of toxins is aided. Endorphins are also released to improve our mood, brain activity is increased, and stress hormones are lowered.

Certain sorts of massage, such as shiatsu, act on the energy meridians in the body, balancing the flow of energy around the whole body.

Massage generally concentrates on working on the muscles to release tension.

Types of massage

There are many different types of massage, from Swedish massage to shiatsu and shen tao, which are based on acupressure. We look at these three specific examples below.

Swedish massage This is the type of massage with which most of us are familiar. It was developed by Per Henrik Ling at the end of the 19th century as a therapeutic massage, but is not specifically a holistic treatment. It involves a stroking movement, called effleurage, a squeezing and kneading stroke called petrissage, a rhythmic tapping stroke using the side of the hand or a cupped hand called tapotement, and friction, which is the pressure applied by the thumbs and knuckles to a knotted muscle. This is not a massage where the therapist will want to know your emotional state, and the effect is short-term. Regular sessions will help keep areas of your body where you hold tension, such as your neck and back, as mobile as possible.

Shiatsu massage This is a whole body massage that originated in Japan early in the 20th century, but it evolved from Traditional Chinese Medicine (TCM). It involves the application of pressure to the acupoints in the body to release the flow of energy using the thumbs, forearms, elbows, knees, and feet to achieve the desired pressure.

Because this is a holistic form of massage, the practitioner may want to know details of your general health and emotional state, as well as your diet and lifestyle. You remain clothed during the massage, unless the practitioner is combining the massage with aromatherapy. It is also suitable for self-application when treating minor ailments such as sinus congestion, headaches, and nausea.

Shiatsu is an energetic, robust massage technique, and it is particularly helpful for depression where the symptoms are mainly lethargy and fatigue, or for stress-related conditions. The treatment itself can sometimes be quite uncomfortable, especially when pressure is applied to an area in your body where tension and blocked energy have accumulated, but the end result is a feeling of relaxation and lifted spirits.

Shen tao This is perhaps one of the oldest forms of acupressure massage, and it is good for depression, stress, and insomnia, but is less vigorous than shiatsu. A whole body therapy based in TCM, it puts pressure on the meridian points using the fingers and hands to restore harmony to the body. Weekly sessions, following a consultation about your symptoms and general health, are usual.

The benefits Massage can be a great comfort, especially to those of us suffering from the isolation of depression. Again, find a therapist who has good credentials and with whom you feel comfortable. A trusting relationship is essential for good results.

Evidence
The Touch Research Institute in Miami, USA, in a study done in 1993, found that girls who were in hospital because they were suffering from eating disorders experienced less anxiety and depression when they were treated with regular massage.

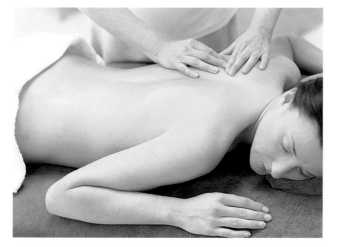

The relaxation and comfort we experience through massage can help us through the dark days of depression.

MASSAGE

Do you feel that you need to be invigorated?

Do you suffer from poor circulation?

Do you want a bit of comfort?

Hydrotherapy

Water is the stuff of life. Our bodies are made up of more than two-thirds water and we also drink it, bathe in it, steam in it, float in it, watch it, and listen to it. It relaxes and heals us, invigorates us, and cleanses us. We can even be born into it these days. How often have you had a stressful day soothed away by a warm, scented bath, or stood under the shower feeling the tension flow out of you in the stream of water?

How it works
There are many different forms of hydrotherapy, but one of water's most important uses is to manipulate the body's blood circulation through the application of hot and cold water. The body responds to heat by the dilation of surface blood vessels, increasing the flow of blood to the skin and muscles, which relaxes the body. When we are hot we sweat and this helps to eliminate toxins from the body. Cold water constricts the surface blood vessels, stimulating the flow of blood to internal organs, and reduces inflammation.

"Taking the waters"
Greeks, Romans, and genteel Victorian ladies all deemed spas necessary for healing and the general maintenance of health. "Taking the waters" in places like Baden-Baden in Germany, or Bath in England, involved drinking and bathing in the mineral-enriched water. Lourdes in France still offers a spring that claims miraculous cures for the incurable.

These days we are more likely to find hydrotherapy at a health farm. The modern equivalent of spas is jacuzzis, which have hot, high-powered water jets that you can direct to areas of muscle tension in your body, or whirlpool baths, in which the pressurized bubbles have the effect of gently pummelling the skin to encourage circulation and promote muscle relaxation. A hydrotherapist might also suggest you brush your skin afterwards with a loofah or skin brush. If you do this, start from your feet, work your way up your body towards your heart, and use firm, circular brushing motions. This will help to eliminate toxins and will also improve your circulation.

Exercising in water Water has the property of buoyancy, which makes it an excellent vehicle for exercise, especially if someone is suffering from muscle injury or tension, because the body is supported, making muscle strain less likely. Water exercises and swimming can be good starting points for someone unused to exercise, and they also have the advantage of being suitable for all ages and states of physical fitness.

Saunas and steam rooms Saunas produce a dry heat, while steam rooms and turkish baths produce a wet steam. All of them make the body sweat to get rid of toxins, relax the muscles, and increase the blood flow around the body. Some people find the harsher heat of a sauna uncomfortable to sit in while others prefer it to the damp blanket heat of a steam room. Try both types to decide which one suits you best, but don't stay in for too long, especially if you are not used to the experience. Get up slowly when you have finished your session, which ideally should be no more than 15 minutes, then take a cold shower, to close up the pores on your skin and clear your head. Drink plenty of water before and after a session as sweating means the loss of body fluids, which need to be replaced. Regular use of steam can help maintain a healthy body system by reducing the build up of waste products accumulated in conditions like depression, which are caused by tension, poor diet, and lack of exercise. After a session you should feel both invigorated and relaxed.

Flotation therapy A flotation tank is not for everyone, and is not a good idea for those who suffer from claustrophobia. However, for many people, flotation therapy induces a deep sense of mental and physical relaxation. Developed in America in the 1970s, the theory behind it is that the weightlessness combined with the absence of external stimuli, which you experience by being immersed in body-temperature water in an enclosed tank, allow complete relaxation of the mind and body. The water contains beneficial mineral salts that also provide buoyancy. (Flotation therapy is normally done in dim light for up to an hour and a half.) Regular flotation sessions can help reduce anxiety and the levels of stress hormones in the body.

The general benefits of water We are liable to think of water as merely something that we use to make us clean, but even soaking in a warm bath does more for us than wash off the dirt. Whatever type of hydrotherapy you may want to try, remember also to use water in all its forms to soothe and relax your body.

Drink it

How much water do you drink every day? Many of us don't drink any, as our fluid intake consists entirely of coffee, tea, fizzy drinks, or alcohol. But as we lose at least one and a half litres of water a day through sweating and excretion, we need to replace what is lost. There is a lot of resistance to the recent trend in buying mineral water instead of drinking what comes from the tap. However, it is a known fact that the average spring water provides, among other minerals, 100mg of calcium per litre, whereas tap water in a soft-water area only provides around 30mg, and can contain harmful nitrates and lead too.

Evidence

An American study carried out in 1996 found that whirlpool baths were effective in reducing the reaction to stress in 85% of the people studied. Still and whirlpool baths were both effective in reducing anxiety.

Do you generally feel weak and tired?

Do you have difficulty sleeping at night?

Do you feel that you need more energy?

Reflexology

Applying pressure to the soles of the feet in the form of foot massage has been popular for centuries, both as a relaxation technique and to promote healing. At the start of the 20th century, the American Dr Fitzgerald developed the theory of "zone therapy", which forms the basis of modern reflexology. It treats blocked energy and stimulates the body's healing response, so can be applied to a range of illnesses.

How it works

According to reflexology the body is divided into 10 vertical zones. This zoning follows the same principle as the acupuncture meridians (see page 84), because it also works on the premise that channels of energy flow through the body, but it does have its own separate system. Each organ in the body is allocated to a zone. Practitioners detect granular deposits, made up of lactic acid, calcium crystals, and uric acid, on the reflex points on the foot correlating to organs that are weak, and it is the breaking down of these deposits that releases the healing energy to bring about relief.

The reflexology map

In the 1930s, the American Eunice Ingham expanded Dr Fitzgerald's zone concept and went on to allocate an exact point on the foot for each area of the body, drawing a map to illustrate her theory. This map is used by reflexologists today. While some people still consider this theory of "reiteration", which states that the body is mirrored on the feet, as very controversial, there is plenty of research that suggests that this modern technique is highly successful.

Ingham's reflex points are not just on the sole of the foot, but are found on the sides and top as well, although the majority are in fact located on the base. The reflex point for the brain, for instance, is located on the tips of each toe while the point for the heart is on the inside edge of the ball of the foot. The hypothalamus, the area of the brain that influences the hormonal system, has a reflex point on the big toe. (See the illustration opposite, bottom right, for further details of these reflex points.)

Because our feet are more sensitive to touch than our hands are, reflexology concentrates on the feet, but there are also reflex points on the hands. These points are used for sinus and intestinal problems, such as irritable bowel syndrome.

Visiting a therapist

As reflexology is a holistic therapy, the therapist will start a session with questions about your general health, although reflexologists do not consider themselves to be trained to comment on your emotional state. They claim their technique does not diagnose medical conditions, nor cure specific ailments, but works on releasing the flow of body energy to activate the healing response and stimulate the circulation to flush out waste products that contribute to ill health. Like practitioners of Traditional Chinese Medicine, reflexologists believe that when energy pathways are free flowing, the body and mind will achieve optimum health themselves.

You will be asked to lie down with your feet uncovered, while the therapist massages your feet to relax them. Thumb walking is the most popular technique therapists in the West use. This involves pressing and releasing the pads of the thumbs in a slow, regular rhythm onto a pressure point. The points that need particular attention will be signalled by tenderness in a specific area. Some therapists believe that outer manifestations, such as hard areas of skin, bunions, and corns are also signs of trouble in the area of the body correlating to the reflex point affected. The therapist will apply pressure to the tender point, kneading it to break down the gritty deposits.

Most people who experience reflexology say that the process can be quite painful at first, depending on the degree of build up of crystals and acids, but subsequent treatments are less painful. After the initial session it is not unusual to develop a slight headache as the toxins start moving out of the organs and into the bloodstream to be eliminated. As with other holistic therapies, one session will probably only have a short-term benefit, so it is better to embark on a course of treatment, depending on your problem, with occasional maintenance sessions.

Providing relaxation Although it seems a strange idea that points on our feet mirror our body organs, this therapy does appear to be effective and, even after just one session, most people find that it has relaxed them as well as helped to alleviate any stress and fatigue they had been experiencing.

Aromatherapy and reflexology

Reflexologists do not use oils while massaging the feet, but some aromatherapists use reflexology to help with their diagnosis. Once they have used the technique to determine the diagnosis, they then select which essential oils should be used in the treatment.

Evidence

A three-year Danish study of 235 postal workers published in 1993 found that 176 of them (that is, 75% of the people studied) reported relief from symptoms such as stress headaches, backache, and neck strain after weekly reflexology sessions. Sick days per employee were generally reduced from 11.4 to 8.5 days per year too.

Selected reflexology areas

brain

lung

stomach
pancreas

small
intestine

sciatic

Do you often feel out of sorts?

Are you particularly susceptible to illness?

Are you emotionally exhausted?

Colour therapy

We all respond subconsciously to the colours around us. We have a favourite colour, know which particular colours suit us, and also make instinctive colour choices for different rooms in our homes. Colour therapy follows the theory that each colour has a vibrational energy that can influence our own body energy to promote relaxation as well as to heal.

How it works

The universe is said to be made up of vibrational energies. These energies all vibrate at different rates, or frequencies, to create light, colour, and sound.
Each colour is said to have a different vibrational frequency – for instance, red vibrates faster than blue. A colour therapist aims to bring the body back to a state of harmony, and therefore into good health, by using the vibrational frequency of colour to rebalance the body's energies.

Auras

We each have a physical body but we also have, according to ancient spiritual wisdom, subtle bodies made of pure energy: the etheric body, astral body, mental body, and spiritual body. Our aura is the collective term for these subtle bodies, which manifest themselves in colours that are invisible to most of us, but can be seen by some spiritual healers. Our auras surround each of us with layers of rainbow colours, and a colour therapist is able to see our aura and can make a diagnosis depending on which colours predominate in which areas.

If we are healthy, our etheric body, the one closest to our physical body, will emit a rainbow glow 10cm (4in) from our body. If we are ill, or are about to become ill, our etheric body might be dull, be too close to the body, and contain dark patches that represent blocked energy. Our astral body is said to be concerned with our emotional health, and is seen as a green oval outside the etheric body. Someone who is suffering from depression might have a dull green, or yellow-green, astral body.

Chakras and colour Chakras, the seven major energy centres of the body defined by ancient Indian spiritual wisdom (see pages 78–9), are each represented by a different colour in the spectrum: red for the base chakra, orange for the sacral chakra, yellow for the one on the solar plexus, green for the heart chakra, blue for the throat chakra, indigo for the one located on the forehead, and violet for the crown chakra (see box, right). When our chakras are out of balance we become ill or susceptible to illness because the flow of subtle energy through the body is blocked. A colour therapist might focus colour onto a particular chakra to restore its balance, either with coloured light or crystals of a specific colour.

Visiting a therapist

There are various ways that a colour therapist can diagnose your condition. Some will simply read your aura to detect any colour imbalances while some may dowse your chakras, holding a crystal pendulum above each one to determine the vibrational energy. Others simply pass coloured cards in front of you and allow you to choose the ones that seem relevant to you.

The therapist will then treat you with coloured light or crystals. You will need to sit or lie down, preferably wearing white so as not to interfere with the colour treatment, for a specific length of time while you are bathed in a light of the most beneficial colour. Indigo is said to calm anxiety and insomnia, violet helps with self-esteem, yellow is good for emotional exhaustion, orange for depression, and blue for melancholy. The therapist might also suggest that you surround yourself with the appropriate colour in your home. To avoid imbalance, the therapist might introduce a secondary colour to complement the dominant one as too much of one colour may affect your health.

Using colour in the home

Everything has a colour, but we often fail to notice the wealth of healing colour around us. Take another look at nature to see the vibrancy of colours, such as a bright blue sky or a ripe red tomato. We can also use our instinct to choose the colours in our home. Don't paint your bedroom red if you have trouble sleeping; it is an energizing colour, so try calming blue instead. If you find cooking a problem, surround yourself with yellow in the kitchen to create balance and self-confidence. Change your black jumper for a violet one when you want to be inspired creatively or spiritually. Use colour to create healing energy and tranquillity.

The seven chakras
Chakras are the major energy centres of the body defined by ancient Indian spiritual wisdom.

Violet : crown

Indigo : forehead

Blue : throat

Green : heart

Yellow : solar plexus

Orange : sacrum

Red : base

Kirlian photography
In 1939 a Russian scientist called Semyon Kirlian discovered a technique for photographing auras. A person's feet or hands are placed on a metal plate covered with light-sensitive paper. The paper is then subjected to a high-voltage current. Practitioners who use this method say that the size, quality, and radiance of the energy field visible on the photograph indicates the state of the person's body energy.

Do you live with uncomfortable noise levels?

Are you often extremely tense?

Do you find it hard to express your feelings?

Music therapy

Sound, like light and colour, has a powerful effect on our emotions. Surrounded by noise, much of it unwelcome and intrusive, it is easy to recognize our negative response to sound. The combination of cars, telephones, and noisy neighbours can send us into a permanent low-level state of tension, even if we are not aware of it. But music and sound can also have a therapeutic effect on us.

How it works

There are many different ways that sound is used. The vibrational energy generated by chanting is said to respond to the body's vibrational energy to bring about the inner harmony of cells, organs, and energy flow. Listening to soothing music is said to lower the heart rate and respiration, and so helps to relieve stress, while stimulating music is said to increase brain activity. The free-form playing of instruments, particularly drums, is a method of energy release and self-expression that can improve our confidence. Our response to the music that we love to listen to, or singing without inhibition, releases mood-enhancing endorphins to raise our spirits.

Music and general sound

We all love music in some form, even if we don't consider ourselves to be musical. We might like country and western music, Beethoven, or the theme tune to our favourite television show, but, whatever our preference is, we subconsciously respond to it and feel pleasure. Like a particular smell, music can also evoke a time, place, person, or emotion acutely. Many of us play music as a background to our lives; in the car, a shop, restaurant, or have the radio on constantly while we work. But we are not really listening to it. When your spirits need a lift, or you are feeling tense, put on a piece of your favourite music and make yourself comfortable. Don't read or talk, just simply sit back and listen to the rhythm and the notes and let yourself be completely taken over by the sound.

Rhythms and chants The use of sound to alter our state of consciousness and promote healing has long been recognized in both religious and spiritual rituals. African and shamanic drumming use a persistent rhythm that continues for hours on end without a break until the listeners are drawn up into the beat. This beating is said to represent the rhythm of life and it corresponds to the beating of the heart. Eventually the vibrational sound causes listeners to lose awareness of the world around them and experience a higher spiritual plane.

Chanting also uses vibrations to create a meditative state and promote spiritual and mental well-being. It has been practised for centuries by Buddhist monks, but has recently become more popular in the West. You do not have to be able to sing in tune to chant. Chanting is often done in groups, and is used by music therapists. Participants might sit in a circle with the therapist who will choose a note to begin. He or she will then teach them to manipulate the note, bringing its vibrations to different areas of their body until they begin to hear not only the note but other notes, or harmonics, which vibrate with the original note to create an extraordinary sound both inside and outside their heads. The note manipulation can be brought about by changing the shape of our mouths, moving our tongues, and breathing into the note. It is difficult to understand how powerful the effect is unless you have tried it, and it is well worth the experience. Feelings of euphoria and a deep sense of peace are often reported after a chanting session. This can be particularly beneficial if you are suffering from anxiety or stress.

Using music therapy The National Association of Music Therapy in North America was set up in the 1950s, closely followed by The British Society of Music Therapy in the late 1950s. The latter now has a music therapy foundation and a therapist's training course. The foundation has become world famous for treating autistic children and those with learning difficulties, but the same sort of therapy is also applied to people with anxiety, depression, and problems with expressing their repressed emotions.

If you decide to try music therapy, here is a description of what you might experience. The therapist will play some music and will then encourage you to join in either by singing or playing an instrument like a drum or cymbal. This does not involve any musical skill, and the music will mostly be improvized. Both the sound and the physical involvement can be cathartic in releasing inhibitions and allowing the expression of feelings. Just singing at the top of your lungs can also create enormous energy.

Sounds that are therapeutic and restful can have a very calming and beneficial effect. Try to include such music in your everyday life to reap some of these benefits.

Evidence
In 1994 a study done at Stanford University School of Medicine, USA took 30 depressed people over 80 years old and divided them into two groups. One group was given weekly music therapy, the other no treatment at all. The music therapy group had less anxiety, distress, and low moods and more self-esteem than the other group.

Sounds of nature
Although most of us spend very little time in our natural environment, we are said to be soothed by natural sounds such as birdsong, flowing water, whales communicating, the sound of waves, and falling rain. Many alternative therapists will play recordings from nature during treatment sessions, and some suggest that this form of sound can be a helpful aid to meditation and relaxation.

Spiritual
thoughts

Organized religion in the West has, in a way, allowed many of us to put our innate spirituality on hold. We have learned to accept the dictates of where, how, and when to worship and what to believe. We are no longer in touch with the vast well of intuition, imagination, and spiritual wisdom that we all possess.

Many of us have also been put off from embarking on our own personal spiritual journey because of the associations that this has with the New Age movement. Many are cynical about it, believing that it is only for candle-wielding hippies and bandwagon phoneys, but they haven't taken the time to examine the ancient teachings and traditions that have inspired the movement.

We have become techies, struggling with the material and technical in our lives while excluding a deeper awareness of who we are, why we are here, and where we are going. But now, more than ever, we have available to us a wealth of information upon which to draw, from spiritual teachings in many different ancient and modern cultures. They allow us to choose how we see God, either as a denominational figure or an areligious spiritual presence.

Without a spiritual dimension to our life, our existence can seem pointless, and, as a result, our emotional and mental health can be affected. Accessing spiritual knowledge can be done through prayer, spiritual texts, or in the more structured surroundings of retreats, ashrams, and communes. Whichever way you choose, you will certainly benefit from the wisdom and insights you will receive.

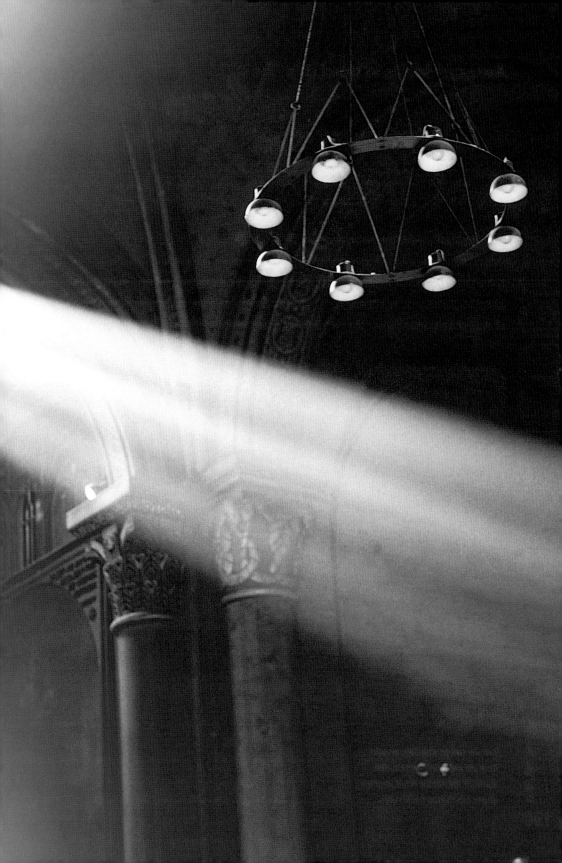

Are your spirits in need of a boost?

Do you suffer from anxious thoughts?

Are you out of touch with nature?

Get back to nature

Getting back to nature somehow conjures up an image of frolicking naked in the woods with garlands of flowers in our hair. However, a closer association with the natural world can offer us healing. Seeing the blossoms of spring, for instance, gives us a sense of continuity and connection to a wider universe. And such things also give us a break from the sometimes tiring manipulations of other human beings.

How it works
Breathing fresh air in deeply, allowing natural light to enter our eyes, and smelling flowers and herbs all create stimulants for the centre in our brain called the hypothalamus, which affects our mood by regulating our hormonal balance.

An urban existence
More of us live in urban, or semi-urban, settings than ever before. There is nothing intrinsically wrong with this, and to romanticize the natural world and say that all of us would be better off living in the countryside is neither practical nor helpful. However, it is important not to lose touch with nature. The cycles of nature are our own cycles, as we are all elements of the same universe. It is only because we have civilized and educated ourselves into the narrow confines of a materialistic world that we see nature as somehow separate to us.

"Finding the silence which contains thoughts, whatever they do they hear the Truth."
Zen saying

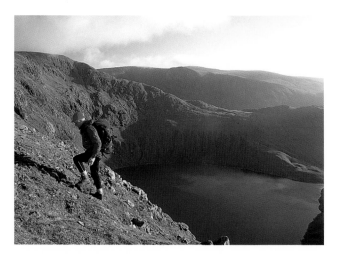

Feel the sun on your face, breathe fresh air, and smell the beautiful scents of the natural world as often as you can to reap the benefits.

130

Traditions of nature

Most religious teachers and spiritual leaders are said to have spent time alone with nature. Jesus spent 40 days in the wilderness; Siddhartha, who became the Buddha, spent six years on a riverbank; and Muhammad saw his visions in a cave. Human interaction, although vital to our happiness, does prevent the possibility of communion with ourselves. We cannot listen to our intuition, acknowledge what we are feeling, or recognize our emotional needs when we are having to listen and respond to others all day long. If we are not careful we can forget how to be alone, and it can then seem frightening and unsafe.

The natural world is a wonderful place in which to be alone. It welcomes us and supports us, offering a perfect setting for meditation and tranquillity. Martial arts such as Tai chi and Qigong are often practised in the open air for this very reason.

Shamanism Native spiritual wisdom, called shamanism, still exists in the indigenous tribes of Africa, Australia, and North America, among others. It centres on the tribes' powerful connection with nature. They see the earth as sacred; the birds, animals, and trees are imbued with spirits, some good, some bad, and they will decorate their dwellings and clothes with images of these animal spirits. Their ritual dancing also mimics the movements of animals. Sacred plants – such as mushrooms – that can have mind-altering properties, are used both in their healing and sacred rituals.

Natural phenomenon

Everything on the earth is affected by lunar cycles, including the tides, women's menstruation cycles, and our propensity for mood swings and depression. Low barometric pressure, wind directions and temperatures, and thunderstorms all leave us vulnerable to mood swings and certain ailments like asthma or rheumatism. The positively charged ions that fill the atmosphere before a thunderstorm also make most of us feel headachy and tense.

We all understand that our children need fresh air, but somehow when we grow up we forget how much we enjoyed the natural world. So follow the children's example and get out a bit more. You will definitely feel better once you have done it.

Refresh yourself

Take some time to be in the natural world. If you are a city dweller, find a garden or a park, and sit on a bench or on the grass for an hour to just feel the presence of nature around you. Go early in the morning or at dusk when it is quiet and listen to the birds, watch the season as it changes, and smell the earth and the flowers. You will be surprised how restful an experience this is and how your spirits will be raised by such moments. It will also help you to clear your mind of anxious thoughts as well as to relax your body.

Try gardening

Gardening has long been recognized as good for the soul. The acts of seeding, weeding, pruning, and watering are seen by some as a metaphor for how we nurture our spirituality. It is also a place where you can express your individual creativity, and have your own private sanctuary. Choose flowers and plants for your garden that not only appeal to you visually, but whose scents also lift your spirits. If you haven't got a garden, plant a window box or tub, or create an indoor garden in a corner of your house. You will soon notice the benefits.

Does your immune system need a boost?

Are you open to the possibilities of healing energy?

Do you harness your own healing powers enough?

Energy healing

For some time now there has been a huge chasm between the Western, conventional, approach to medicine and the system of traditional Eastern healing. Western medicine uses scientific methods to treat specific conditions that are thought to develop for no particular reason. Eastern healing focuses mainly on the realignment and freeing up of body energy, and takes a holistic approach that involves the mind, body, and spirit.

How it works

There are many different healing philosophies, but they all rely on the same principle of channelling the healing power of some higher spirit through the healer and into the recipient, to rebalance the body energies and stimulate the immune system to begin the process of healing the body.

Subconscious healing

It is said that we all have the power to heal, but don't use it. However, most of us will have experienced a moment when we did. It may have been when we developed the start of a cold, but because we had a big day coming up and couldn't be ill, we told the cold to go away, and it did – we subconsciously activated our healing powers.

Using healing energy

People who are able to focus their energy into healing often combine this skill with other techniques such as cranial osteopathy, aromatherapy, and shiatsu – any therapy where the practitioner's hands are placed on or near the patient's body. The therapists may not be able to say where their energy comes from, but most believe they are tapping into a universal energy.

When the healing energy is generated, a warmth comes off the healer's hands, and this has been accessed through concentration or meditation. Some healers place their hands directly on the patient's body, while others deal with the aura, or energy field, around the body, so their hands hover slightly away from it. All conditions are said to be helped by energy healing, as it treats the body's energy, not the actual symptoms of illness.

Crystals may also be used by healers, as they are known to contain healing properties. The healer places the relevant crystal on the chakras (see pages 78 and 125) of the patient's body. For example, they may place an amethyst on the forehead to quieten the mind.

Different forms of spiritual healing

Spiritual healing is, specifically, the channelling of divine energy through a medium into the sick person, so that the patient's healing powers can be stimulated. All religions have healers, such as shamans or priests, but there are also healers who do not believe in a denominational god, but in a wider definition of a divine spiritual presence. Some people refer to spiritual healing as the "laying on of hands". A practitioner will do just that, lay their hands on the person to be healed. It does need the recipient to believe that it will work – without their faith it won't (see box, right). This also applies to faith healers, who believe that the ill person will only be healed if they have faith in whichever particular god the healer is representing. You obviously have to be careful when choosing a healer, as there are charlatans who prey on vulnerable people, so take time to find a reputable one.

Spiritualist healing Spiritualists believe that they can summon up spirits from the spirit world who have healing powers that they themselves do not possess. The spiritualist will go into a trance in order to connect with the relevant spirit.

Absent healing This form of healing does not require the healer and the recipient to be in the same place. The healer will meditate or pray for the patient, sending healing energies without bodily contact. Nuns or monks in closed orders will often use this sort of distance healing through prayer.

Radionics is a form of absent healing that uses physical "witnesses", ie a sample of hair or handwriting from the patient, from which the practitioner dowses (using a pendulum) the energy imbalances and decides on the potential remedies, such as homeopathic or herbal preparations.

Reiki This is a healing art that originated in Japan in the 19th century, and it has its roots in Tibetan Buddhism. During Reiki, the practitioner channels healing energies from higher spiritual planes into the client through the laying on of hands. Beyond healing the presenting problem, Reiki also seeks to help a client achieve a higher state of consciousness. It is practised with the client clothed and the practitioner places his or her hands on various points on the body where the energy seems to be blocked. This technique can engender a feeling of deep inner peace and joy as well as bodily relaxation.

The placebo effect

This is the rationale used by sceptics for why spiritual energy healing is sometimes seen to be effective. Conventional medicine uses placebos (pills or treatments that are actually useless, for instance sugar pills that contain no active drug) in drug-testing trials. This is to test how much of the drug's performance is due to the expectation of the patient that it will work. But no one can actually explain why a high percentage of those on the placebo do as well as those taking the real drugs. It is clear that what the mind believes to be true has a powerful impact on the body, and this is probably also an important part of spiritual healing.

Evidence

A British trial carried out in 1986 divided 60 patients with tension headaches into two groups. One group was treated with spiritual healing, while the other group was given a placebo treatment. Patients given the spiritual healing had a much better, longer lasting, relief from pain than the other group experienced.

Do you feel that you need a break?

Are you looking for a specific type of spiritual guidance?

Do you long for a bit of peace and quiet?

Retreats

Many Western nations have moved away from the habit of regular church attendance. So where do we go to find instruction in religion and spirituality? Retreats, both religious and non-religious, have become increasingly popular. In fact, there are now themed retreats such as garden retreats, icon painting, and journalling retreats. You can also get involved in activities that encourage self-discovery and spiritual insight.

How it works

How many of us go on holiday for a rest, only to come back totally exhausted due to the travelling, the strange food, sunburn, and the rushing about we did to ensure we got value for money? Retreats provide an alternative to this – a real opportunity to wind down. They are usually set in very tranquil surroundings, and the programme is designed to include times for silence and solitude. If troubled by emotional problems or a crisis of the spirit, you will be able to talk to someone familiar about such dilemmas, or can simply obtain general spiritual guidance. If you are interested in a particular philosophy, this is an ideal way to learn the basics. Many people go on regular retreats once or twice a year just to relax and refresh their spirit.

Who goes on retreats?

The impression most of us have of those who go on retreats is of earnest, sandal-wearing vegetarians who are thrilled by the prospect of sleeping in dormitories and getting up at 5am to meditate. However, these days a huge range of people use various types of retreat to recharge their batteries. Old and young and rich and poor can all be found at retreats, and the only connection between them is their desire to take a spiritual journey. The retreat that you choose for yourself will reflect the things in which you are interested, and the people you will meet once there will all have a similar goal to you.

Retreats are places where we can reflect on our lives. If we are feeling mentally and spiritually exhausted then they can offer a space in which to begin to understand ourselves better, to realize why we are so stressed by our normal lives, and to teach us techniques and philosophies to make us able to cope better.

We spend so much time surrounded by noise, work, and people that it can be quite difficult at first to accept silence and solitude, or the disciplines of meditation. The absence of outside stimuli to distract us from ourselves means that we have to acknowledge an interior existence, and initially we may panic and think that we don't have one, or are scared of what we

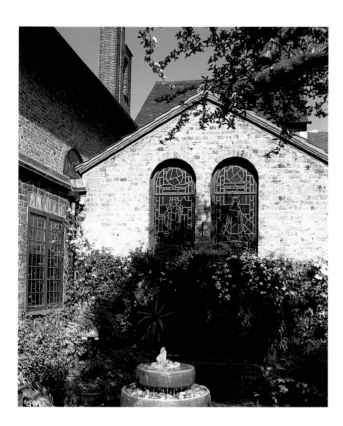

Retreats come in all shapes and sizes, but they are always places of tranquillity, away from noise and the pressures of life.

might discover. You may also find being in a group quite difficult to get used to and may experience irritation with your fellow retreaters, or feelings of insecurity that everyone else is more spiritually enlightened than you are.

The great thing about a retreat is that you are allowed to feel these things, talk about them, and understand what they mean. There should be someone there who is able to interpret a part of the vast lexicon of spiritual and religious teachings from men and women throughout history who have gone through the same sort of spiritual crises as you.

Retreats are not psychotherapy sessions, and, although there is often one-to-one spiritual guidance on offer, they are mainly places for the examination of our spiritual lives. Retreats can be not only a wonderful break, but also may be a jumping off point for a spiritual journey and many people return to them on a regular basis, not just when they are feeling low or exhausted.

Do you want to begin a spiritual journey?

Are you ready to be released from past anger?

Do you want to calm your mind?

Spiritual disciplines

There are many exercises, rituals, and practices attached to spiritual traditions that are intended to help us find ways into our inner consciousness. Ones that you will be familiar with include meditation, Tai chi, and yoga. There are others that may seem more esoteric, but you might actually find that they are just right for you, such as fasting or contemplation. Use your intuition to choose the one for you.

How it works

Spiritual practices are not about notching up points for a spiritual merit badge. They are a means to an end, and that end is personal spiritual growth and enlightenment. It is easy to think that if we are constantly doing spiritual things then we will automatically become spiritual. But it won't work unless we focus on our final aim rather than trying to perfect the practice. The Zen masters tell us that we are already perfect, and that the purpose of spiritual practice is to understand that fact. They say that we should let the discipline come to us, and only do it when it feels right. Let it happen and then let it go.

Deciding on your quest

Many of us get trapped all too easily into habits and routines that make us unhappy. We can't relax, do too much, fall out with friends, or pursue a career that we don't enjoy. We often just don't realize that we can actually change our lives. The changes don't have to be dramatic, external changes such as dumping our job or our partner – they can be changes to our inner self that give us the strength and understanding to make our lives work better for us.

Before you embark on any spiritual practice, decide what it is that you are looking for. Do you really want to begin a spiritual journey, or simply want to calm your mind, let go of past anger, or perhaps just be happier? Do you want to seek guidance from a teacher, a group, or try some things for yourself? Are you prepared to give the practices you choose some regular time? Start small, be open to suggestions, read about what is on offer, and you will quickly find something that seems right for you.

Daily meditations A good place to start your spiritual practice is with a book of meditations. These books offer the background to a spiritual philosophy while being easier to manage than dense scriptural texts. They also contain concepts for living a more fulfilling life within them.

The Dalai Lama, the exiled spiritual and political leader of the Tibetan people, thinks that cultivating a positive state of mind is the key to finding happiness and serenity. His book, *The Path to Tranquillity*, is a compilation of his thoughts and provides one for each day of the year (see box, right, for an example).

Fasting This is practised by every religion and spiritual tradition and is said to rid the body of impurities, strengthen will power, and also leave the mind clear for spiritual thoughts. Find a day when you don't have to work or socialize, unless those you are meeting are also fasting. Drink lots of mineral water all day, keep warm, and rest or take gentle exercise, such as yoga or a walk in the fresh air. Try not to be around other peoples' food, as it makes it too hard if you are not experienced. Beginners could start with drinking fruit juice instead of water as this is more substantial and has some calories. You may feel light-headed or experience headaches at first but it will get easier if you persevere. If fasting is a practice you enjoy, you can slightly increase the length of time you do it for when you next fast.

Fire ceremony This is a ritual for ridding ourselves of patterns of thoughts and feelings that are stopping our spiritual growth.

1 Write down whatever feelings you are uncomfortable with. For instance, you might be fed up with feeling inferior to everyone around you. You could write, "I no longer want to think everyone else is looking down on me".
2 Light a candle and place it in a fireproof container (such as a roasting tin or metal wastepaper bin), or make a fire outside if possible. You can do this exercise with friends if you like.
3 Say goodbye to your bad feeling as you light your paper with the candle and drop it into the container to burn, or simply throw your paper into the flames. Watch the paper being consumed by the fire. This symbolic burning of an unwanted thought can be the trigger for real progress.

Whatever spiritual discipline you choose, try to see it as a doorway to your spirituality, rather than merely a temporary cure for a problem. This way the practice will also help you with the ongoing development of your spiritual understanding.

"Human potential is the same for all. Your feeling, 'I am of no value' is wrong. Absolutely wrong. You are deceiving yourself. We all have the power of thought – so what are you lacking? If you have will power, then you can do anything. It is usually said that you are your own master."
Dalai Lama

Do you need time for reflection?

Do you need to be reminded of your intuitive powers?

Do you seek spiritual inspiration?

Journalling

Keeping a diary is a way of focusing our thoughts and keeping a record of the ups and downs of our existence. Journalling is the spiritual equivalent, the recording of the events that take place in our inner life in order to have a better understanding of our progress along the spiritual path. It also gives us a chance to realize how much the divine is actually present in our lives.

How it works

Most of us don't have a lot of time to reflect on our lives, as we are too busy living them. Events come and go and it is hard to get any real perspective on what happened, or what it has meant to us. If we embark on a spiritual journey it helps to mark down the moments as they occur, even if at the time we have no chance to contemplate their meaning.

Seeing things more clearly

Set a time aside every day, perhaps at night when events are still fresh in your mind, to jot down thoughts, intuitions, times when you felt a prayer or question was answered, or times when you received special help from an outside source. Use a book that is solid and beautiful so that you will enjoy writing in it. At first you will probably think that what you are writing is just a pile of ramblings but gradually, if you keep up the practice, a pattern will emerge from among it all. For instance, if you are recording times when you feel spiritually low, when everything is going wrong, and there seems to be no help available, reflecting on past times when you have felt this way can help you discover why it happens. It could be because you are with people who are spiritually draining for you, or you might be repeating mean-spirited or angry behaviour that is being reflected back in the way others treat you. You might, therefore, find that you have been blaming others when you were just as much to blame.

Alternatively, reading your journal might make you realize just how much divine help you are receiving. Perhaps there is a day when you send up a prayer for help in completing a piece of work you are having trouble understanding. A small miracle perhaps, but such help seems to come out of the blue. It is easy to miss these incidents unless you keep a record of them.

Journalling also helps us with our intuition. How many times have you known that you should not go to a particular place, meet a particular person, or make a particular decision, and you have been proved right? This is not just hindsight, an inner voice will have told you, but often we don't recognize or remember it. By writing these incidents down it will remind us of the opportunities that we missed, any intuition that we ignored, and will also focus our attentions on finding the spiritual dimension to our lives. Take time once a week to review what you have written and make a note of the predominant impressions of the week. For instance you might decide that there were too many occasions when you didn't stand up for what you believed to be right. Don't blame yourself – just become aware of what you are doing and you will then be ready to make any necessary changes.

Writing down your spiritual practices Once you decide on your spiritual goal, or the discipline you intend to practice, it often helps to write it down. We can have all sorts of intentions, many of which are unrealistic, but somehow writing them down separates the possible from the ridiculous. For instance, it would be great to meditate for two hours a day but with three children, a full-time job, and no partner, this plan is doomed to failure. Write down your goals for the next week and then at the end of that week, see how you have done and adjust the following week's intentions accordingly. Perhaps, for example, meditating for 20 minutes three times a week would work better.

Lives of inspirational people Reading the thoughts of spiritual teachers can be inspiring because we realize that they had all the same doubts, vanities, and desires that we have. Mahatma Gandhi, Zen master Thich Nhat Hanh, St Augustine, the Dalai Lama, Taoist philosopher Lao Tzu, who wrote the *Tao Te Ching*, and Sufi poets and sages such as Rabi'a and the Prophet Kahlil Gibran have all written with great humanity and accessibility. Or, if you prefer, read our modern gurus such as M Scott Peck, Sai Baba, Parmatiansa Yogananda, and Deepak Chopra.

Persevere Writing our thoughts and feelings down regularly can pinpoint areas we need to work on, but can also encourage us when we look back on the things we've come through.

> *"Persons can be found who are good, very good indeed, in fact great… And yet these very same people can at times be boring, irritating, petulant, selfish, angry and depressed. To avoid disillusionment with human nature, we must first give up our illusions about it."*
> Abraham Maslow, psychologist

Are you tired of living in a materialistic world?

Do you want to try a new way of life?

Does your spirit need refreshing?

Communes

Sometimes we need to take a break from our normal routine and immerse ourselves in a spiritual community to fully absorb the teachings of a spiritual leader or religion. Or perhaps we just want to try an alternative lifestyle; the hippies of the 1960s started the vogue for commune living in the West, and the New Age movement has made visiting ashrams in India a popular way of starting a spiritual journey and refreshing our spirits.

How it works

Finding others who support you in your spiritual journey is not always easy, particularly at the outset. But by locating a teacher whose philosophy interests you, or by attending spiritual workshops, you will find like-minded people. It does seem to be true that we are drawn to those who will help us when the time is right, and spending time in a commune is a good way to immerse yourself in a spiritual way of life without the routines of your normal life distracting you.

Simple commune life

Communes are mainly for those of us who want to experience a way of living that eschews materialism. New Agers do this, and usually follow a philosophy based on ecologically sound principles. This means growing organic food free from pesticides and chemicals, recycling waste products, using natural materials for clothing, and conserving energy wherever they can. Most of these communities finance their lifestyle by making craft products, marketing organic fruit and vegetables, and/or holding workshops where they teach alternative therapies. Some communes do have a basis in religion, but many have adopted the vaguer spiritual tenets of the New Age movement.

Although the idea of living a lifestyle that is not led by a desire to be rich and successful is appealing to many of us, it would be a mistake to think that this is an easy option. The same constraints of normal society apply, such as dominant egos, competitiveness, personality clashes, and rivalry. And creature comforts can be in short supply. Central heating might seem a horribly bourgeois invention, but in practice most of us have got used to it, as well as the instant heat of a stove and the flushing of a toilet.

Ashrams There are hundreds of ashrams, which are Hindu-based spiritual communities, all over India, along with a host of different gurus based at these ashrams. Some of the ashrams are extremely basic – people sleep in bare cells, rise before dawn for group meditation, and are given work and a small amount of simple food. But others are more like celestial cities, with facilities to match those of many package holidays. Most expect participants to adhere to the disciplines of the ashram, which might involve such things as work-sharing, fasting, abstinence from sexual activity and the use of alcohol and drugs, and attendance at group meditation or prayer.

Finding an ashram that will suit your specific needs and requirements may take time but it is important to research the facilities, listen to recommendations, and to be realistic when choosing one. Remember, your body doesn't necessarily have to be subjected to deprivation in order for your soul to be enhanced.

Cults Unfortunately religion and spirituality lend themselves to the creation of cults. Because those of us who are seeking spiritual guidance are often going through difficult transitions in our lives, we are particularly vulnerable to a person or group that offers a powerful, alternative life philosophy. There is usually nothing threatening about this – after all Jesus offered just such an opportunity to his followers. A spiritual movement becomes a cult when it adopts a dogmatic, controlling, and exclusive approach to its belief system, and requires a follower to be cut off from people they love in their mainstream life. There have been many examples of cults where this authoritarian vision has ended in terrible tragedy, such as the Waco massacre in Texas, USA in 1993 and the Jonestown massacre in Guyana, West Africa in 1978, when 900 followers of the Reverend Jim Jones died. Not all cults result in the death of their followers, but even so they are best avoided. Don't be taken in by the fact that a group claims to be aligned to a familiar spiritual tradition or religion, as it might still be a cult. Be very careful when choosing a group to join.

Refresh your spirit Low mood states can make us question our lifestyle and beliefs. Taking time in a spiritual community can be a good way to refresh our spirits and offer us mechanisms for dealing more successfully with our future. You could call it a "holiday for the soul".

Prashanthi Nilayam
One of the largest and most famous ashrams is Prashanthi Nilayam, or "Abode of divine peace", which was founded by Sathya Sai Baba in his home village of Puttaparthy in India. Puttaparthy used to be a small village, but it is now growing into a city that millions of spiritual pilgrims visit every year. The main ashram was built in 1950, but there are many other temples now too. People go there to listen to teachings from Sai Baba and his disciples, but also to learn meditation and to find their own spiritual path.

Do you question the point of your existence?

Do you lack a divine presence in your life?

Do you seek self-knowledge?

Religion and prayer

Belief in a higher power is good for us. It gives us a philosophy for life that helps us understand the huge questions that face every human being, such as the reason for our existence, as well as providing guidelines for how we should live a useful and fulfilling life. Even if we no longer attend church regularly, most of us have been brought up in a society that espouses the morals and beliefs outlined by its religion.

How it works

Having a system of belief, even if it is not from an organized religion, gives us somewhere to turn to when our lives confuse us. Without a belief in a higher power many of us lose a sense of purpose, and find our existence empty. Sharing a belief is a form of intimacy and social integration that has been shown to enhance our immune function and so strengthen our resistance to disease.

Prayer

We all pray. We may not get down on our knees and pray to a denominational God but, unconsciously, most of us ask for help at one time or another. Whether it is programming, or an instinctive human reaction, it is hard for most of us not to believe in something greater than ourselves, a universal presence that we can call upon in times of trouble. We seem to have an instinctive knowledge of a divine presence.

Prayer can be performed in groups or alone, silently or out loud, in a holy place or wherever we are when the mood takes us. It is not just about asking for help, it is a way of connecting both with God and with each other. Although meditation has Eastern spiritual connotations, most forms of prayer are meditations – the stilling of the mind to exclude earthly thoughts and concentrate on communing with a higher consciousness.

We don't have to belong to a specific religion to read and understand their prayers. All prayers have a universal context and aim, to be at one with God. So take a broad view, investigate prayer books from different religious traditions, and see what speaks to you. It might be a Christian prayer, a Sufi poem, a passage from the Jewish *Cabala*, a Buddhist mantra, a Celtic myth, or a prayer written by a modern spiritual guru.

When you have found one that appeals to you, listen to the words until you become absorbed in their meaning. Prayers that you become really familiar with and that you love can be of great comfort to you when you are feeling distressed or low.

A new way

The religion we were brought up with is such an intrinsic part of us, even if we no longer practise it, that it seems impossible to change to another belief structure. And if the philosophies of the major religions are broadly similar – Mahatma Gandhi called them "different roads converging on the same point" – then why bother? The ultimate aim to be at one with God might be the same, but each tradition has its own path to this goal, and another way from the one in which you were raised might be more appealing to you as an adult. Investigating other beliefs does not require you to become a card-carrying member of that discipline, but it can renew your spiritual enthusiasm and set you back on a spiritual path.

Praying is very simple. Whether we are kneeling beside our bed at night, as some of us did as children, or are sitting in a packed cathedral, we can all close our eyes and connect with something greater and more powerful than ourselves. Whether we are asking for help or giving thanks for our blessings, prayer is a comforting ritual that gives us a sense of belonging.

Using rituals

Ritual, if performed with thought and sincerity, can be very comforting. Don't be bound by formal worship. If you are feeling low, slip into a beautiful church and say a prayer, or light a candle. You could, alternatively, create a personal shrine in a corner of your house where you can be alone to perform your chosen spiritual rituals.

Evidence

Research done in 1995 at the Dartmouth Medical School in America showed that people with faith were three times more likely to survive open-heart surgery than those without a faith were. It was also shown that it is the feeling of belonging that such a shared faith brings, whether it be political or spiritual, as much as the belief itself, which is the major factor in making us feel more positive about life.

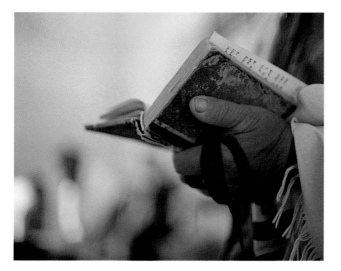

Reading a religious or spiritual text gives us the comfort of being at one with a long tradition of spiritual wisdom and understanding.

Releasing
the mind

Times have changed. These days we can all have the opportunity to express our feelings more openly if we need to. This is good news as being open is very necessary for our well-being – bottling up anger, resentment, and unhappiness causes stress to all the mind and body systems. If we do this our stress-hormones build up and create long-term damage to body organs, but, perhaps more importantly, if we do not talk about how we feel, and don't shout, laugh, and cry when the need arises, then we are less likely to get a healthy perspective on our problems.

In the West, a lot of us still seem to be caught between the traditional "stiff upper lip" of the past – shouldering our emotional burdens silently and without complaint – and the recent frenzy for telling our innermost secrets to perfect strangers on television. The indiscriminate airing of emotional baggage might not necessarily be helpful unless it also elicits an informed response, but neither is it helpful for a person to repress their negative feelings, as this can result in physical and mental ill health. It's a bit like cramming more and more things into an already full bag. In the end something has to give, and in human beings the result of doing this can be depression.

Learning techniques that release the mind from pent-up, uncomfortable, emotions, as well as encouraging free expression, can lead to a much healthier life for every part of us – our minds, our bodies, and our spirits.

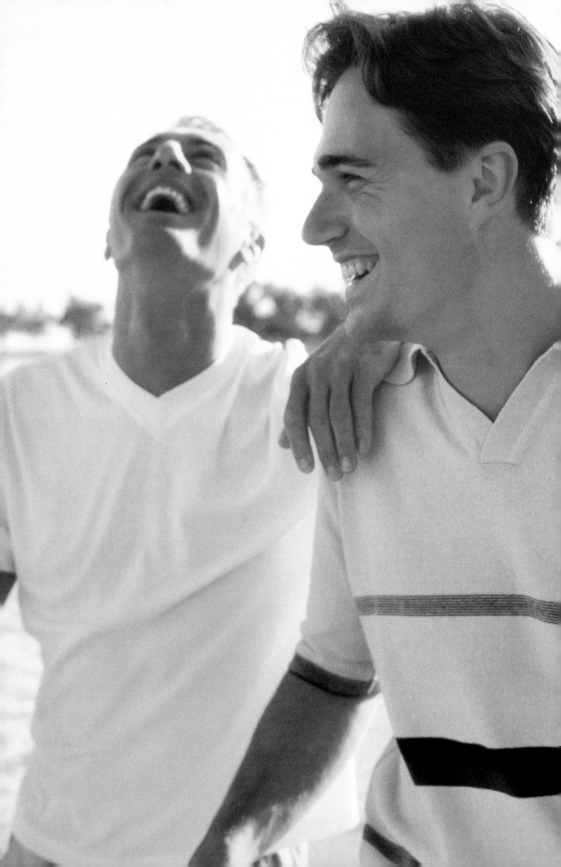

Do you feel that no one listens to you?

Do you often feel isolated and alone?

Do you find it difficult to ask for help?

Talking about it

Talking is an important form of communication but when we get depressed it is often one of the first areas of our lives that we shut down. But talking about our problems to friends, family, or even a trained counsellor can make us feel less isolated and sometimes shed light on why we are depressed. It is therefore extremely important to talk to those around you and tell them how you feel.

How it works

The more isolated we become in our cocoon of depression, the more we cut ourselves off from the potential avenues of help. Telling someone how we feel also focuses our own minds on our situation, and often exposes just how miserable we really are. This realization can be the all-important first step in the healing process.

Communication

Although you can't walk down a street, sit on a bus, or relax in a café these days without being surrounded by people chatting away on their mobile phones, modern technology does not actually promote face to face interaction. Many of us eat our meals in front of the television instead of sitting round the table and talking. We leave messages on answer machines instead of talking directly to each other, get information from the Internet, and send emails instead of telephoning our friends. It is quite possible to spend the day communicating without seeing

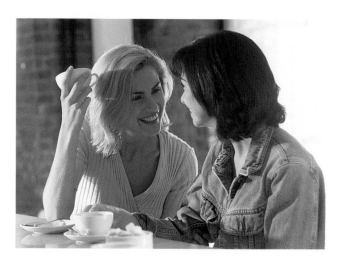

Ring up a friend and arrange to meet for a chat. Just sharing your woes can make them seem more bearable.

another human face. However, the personal, physical interaction between two people is not only a more complete and satisfying way to swap information, it is also a very comforting way to communicate our feelings, especially if we are feeling low.

We can tell a lot from the way a person looks and holds themselves, and from seeing their facial expression. We might ring and ask a friend how they are and they answer that they are fine, as many depressed people do. We can't see that they look pale and perhaps aren't bothering about the way they look.

If you are feeling low, get in touch with someone you trust and ask them to drop round, or go to their house. Alternatively, you could make an appointment to talk to your doctor. Be brave and tell them what is on your mind. Even if you don't know quite what the problem is, tell them how you are feeling. The act of airing your problem, and perhaps admitting you feel depressed, will not only help you to focus on how you really feel, it can also begin the process of asking for help.

Outside help We are sometimes worried that the black thoughts depression can produce are too nasty to speak about to our friends. We think that by revealing these thoughts to them they will think less of us. We may also worry that they will tell others. It is at times like these that it is helpful to talk to a professional. You might not feel ready to have therapy, but an organization such as the UK- and USA-based Samaritans has trained counsellors who will understand and not think it odd that you are feeling the way you are. You can ring them day or night so they are a useful first port of call when you are overwhelmed by depression.

Counselling Counsellors are not trained to probe deeply into the possible reasons for your unhappiness. They will, however, be a sounding board for your thoughts and feelings. Having such a trained and sympathetic ear to listen to your problems can be very therapeutic when you are feeling depressed. It is also useful for someone to offer a wider, more objective perspective to help you gain insight into your emotional state. They will help clarify problems and issues in your life as well as provide that safe and discreet place in which you can open up and talk.

Gestalt therapy

This therapy was developed after World War II by the German psychologist Fritz Perls (1893–1970). The therapy works on the premise that a person's inability to integrate the parts of his or her personality into a healthy whole lies at the root of psychological disturbance. The therapy focuses on the person's behaviour in the here and now, and they are encouraged to express any feelings they may be repressing, often through acting out scenarios.

Opening up

Left to ourselves, we are all capable of blowing up worries and painful feelings in our mind until they assume enormous proportions. But then we tell a friend and suddenly we can laugh about them, or at least find a rational perspective. Depression doesn't go away straight after a chat to a friend, but it helps to know that others understand, and we may also find that many of our friends, perhaps unbeknown to us, have also suffered in the same way.

Is it difficult for you to let go of painful emotions?

Have you lost touch with your creative side?

Do you find it hard to touch and be close to others?

Physical release

In order to release our minds, it can help to release our bodies, as a stiff body often results in a stiff mind. We learn, as we get older, to control our physical movements and to express ourselves verbally, not physically. There is nothing wrong with this but letting go of painful emotions is often not easy, and using energetic movements that take us out of our trained physical probity can help to release our minds.

How it works
If we are having problems articulating painful emotions because we are too scared of letting go, we can turn to an activity that side-steps the psychological process and allows the emotions to be released in a physical way. This makes them seem safer and easier for our mind to acknowledge and understand.

How often do we touch one another?
In 1966 British psychologist Sidney Jourard observed how often couples casually touched each other in an hour. In Paris it was 110 times per hour. In America, twice. In London, zero.

Different approaches

Touch and movement are common to us all, so we don't have to be experts to use physical movements in this way. And there are lots of different approaches to losing your inhibitions without having to rush onto the dance floor and tango. Start small and experiment with something physical that allows you, even momentarily, to let go. Skip down the street, stamp on a pile of leaves, and try to remember what it was like to be a child.

Dance Rhythmic movement, especially that done to the beat of music, or just drums, is especially freeing for the mind. It has been an integral part of many spiritual rituals for centuries, from American Indian rain dancing and African tribal dancing to shamanic ceremonies, where trance is induced with drumming. The Whirling Dervishes, who belong to the Islamic religious sect called Sufis, use sacred dance to induce a trance-like euphoria until they collapse in complete union with God.

When we are dancing we become so absorbed by the instinctive movement of our bodies that we stop thinking. Allowing our conscious thoughts to have a rest also gives our unconscious emotions a chance to be expressed. Young people recognize this freedom, and often lose themselves in physical expression to loud music, but as we get older we tend to forget the youthful knack of being so uninhibited. If you don't feel confident enough to join a dance group or class, find a time when you are alone then put on some music and just move to the rhythm. Be as uninhibited as you like. You might feel silly at first, but you will soon find that the free movement of your body can be exhilarating, and is an excellent way to release pent-up emotions.

Bashing a cushion Anger can be very frightening, not only for the person on the receiving end, but also for the person experiencing the emotion. Anger wells up through our bodies from our guts, and giving vent to it can sometimes seem overwhelmingly destructive. However, you may not have the chance to tell the person who has hurt you or let you down how angry you are, and if that anger is allowed to fester without expression, it can have a detrimental effect on your emotional and physical health, raising your stress hormones and your blood pressure and increasing the likelihood that you will direct your repressed feelings at someone who does not deserve them.

One way of venting your anger, which is now often used in therapy sessions and workshops dealing directly with releasing anger, is to use a rubber or foam baton to beat a cushion or pillow. The cushion symbolizes the person or situation that you are angry with. The release of emotions can be quite extreme with this technique. The person wielding the baton can use as much force as he or she likes and often screams and cries while hitting the cushion. Having a safe, physical outlet for the frustration of repressed anger is said to be very calming and beneficial for those taking part. It is certainly better than kicking the television at home.

Learning how to be intimate Shutting ourselves away in our separate boxes, especially when we are depressed, can mean we have no one to express our emotions to. Talking to each other is vital for emotional health, but touch is also important.

Think about how much physical contact you have with those around you. Do you give and receive hugs or touch your friends as a means of telling them how you feel? Do you hold hands regularly with your partner and/or children? Do you feel very

Dance therapy

Dance therapy, during which the therapist encourages the person to express an uncomfortable emotion through dance and so become more at ease with it, has been popular in America since World War II. Although it is most often used to help disabled people become physically confident, it also has implications for people suffering from low mood states, as they can use the movement as a less confrontational means of airing painful emotions.

comfortable sitting close to others? Try to use physical as well as verbal contact to connect with those around you and make it a channel for expressing your emotions.

Have a good cry We hate seeing someone else cry. It's difficult to watch their raw emotions and to see their pain. So we often stop ourselves from crying because we feel foolish, are nervous about how those around us will react, or worry that if we start crying we won't be able to stop. When something traumatic occurs, if we hold back and don't allow the tears to flow, unexpressed emotions can build up; this bottled up sadness is often one of the contributory causes of depression.

If we don't cry at the time a trauma happens then subsequent, lesser, incidents of loss can take on an unmerited significance. It can also be hard to get in touch later on with the emotion we have buried. We might need to visit the grave of a loved one to be able to cry but, when we have found the trigger for our tears, the most important thing is to give ourselves permission to cry. Tell yourself you are allowed to cry whenever you want to. When you feel the tears coming, don't hold them back. Find some time when you can be alone and cry as hard and as long as you want to. You might spend a whole weekend crying, or cry every night for a week, but you will feel a lot better afterwards. And make sure that you don't bottle up your feelings next time.

Rebirthing This technique, which has recently found popularity with practitioners of New Age therapies, is said to help you release long-held fears and emotions, as well as relive early traumas that you have suppressed. You are able to reach these buried emotions through deep breathing and relaxation techniques carried out in the presence of an experienced therapist. However, the emotions released can be painful and difficult to deal with, so make sure you are confident and comfortable with your practitioner before you start.

Art therapy Many of us lose touch with our creative side once we grow up and take jobs that focus on our managerial, intellectual, administrative, or physical skills. We see painting, drawing, and clay work, unless we are working artists, as child's play and not appropriate now we are adults. But art is very expressive, and art therapy is used as a means of emotional release for anyone who finds talking about problems difficult.

An art therapist will encourage their client to draw, paint, or work with clay – if you undertake such therapy you will be able to choose your own medium. Just the process of free-style creation is cathartic; the smell, feel, colour, and shapes of the materials you use are all an important part of the experience. You are not expected to come up with a fine piece of art, but the results of your work can then be interpreted by the therapist. For instance, you may have drawn yourself, unconsciously, as small and dark and alone beside a group of large, colourful people. Recognizing how you see yourself can help with your self-awareness. Some therapists attach symbolic meaning to certain colours or images, in a similar way to dream symbolism (see page 97), but the insights that spring from art therapy are initiated by the client – the therapist's role is purely that of interpreter.

Psychodrama and role-playing This form of therapy, developed by Austrian psychoanalyst Jacob Moreno in the 1920s, uses drama to act out difficult emotions. Distancing yourself from a problem by role-playing gives you the opportunity to explore and understand how you are feeling without the immediacy of personal confrontation. Once you are familiar with your feelings in the drama, you will be more comfortable with them in reality.

Usually done in workshops over a day or weekend, role-playing is carried out in groups, and each person has a chance to choose a situation they feel uncomfortable with, either from the present or past, and then they act it out with the group. The strong feelings the dramas evoke are then discussed and interpreted by the therapist and the members of the group. This form of therapy can be very helpful if a person has trouble interacting with people in their normal lives because of past trauma.

Finding your way Whether it is talking, touching, dancing, drama, or art, discover the way that helps you express how you feel the best. The more you practise it the easier it will become and the better you will feel in your mind, body, and spirit.

Evidence

Testimonial of a person who successfully worked through depression using art therapy: "Art therapy enables me to access images that no amount of talking can bring to me. It helps me gain a far greater understanding of myself and is a way of expressing painful feelings that until now have had no voice. My painting of black and red figures with daggers is about feeling deeply hurt. The red means pain, the black numbness and death".

Do you have irrational fears?

Does fear stop you from enjoying your life?

Are you afraid that you are actually unlovable?

Banishing fear

Living with a sensible level of fear, such as the fear that prevents us from walking down dark alleys late at night, is normal and part of our survival instinct. Fears about death, old age, or illness are rational fears that we learn to accept as part of life, but the fear of spiders, flying, open spaces, or the fear that comes from low self-esteem is usually less rational, and can be isolating and depressing for the sufferer.

How it works
Facing up to, and getting rid of, the sort of fear that stops us from functioning well, be it phobias or fear of personal inadequacy, make us happier, less prone to low moods, and more able to enjoy a full life.

Unhelpful fear

Self-esteem is developed in childhood. If we are loved and respected for who we are as children, our fears as adults will tend just to be the normal reactions to a challenge or threat. But if we lack self-esteem, the world can be a frightening place. Even walking into a room full of people, having supper with friends, or starting a new relationship can be such a fearful experience that we become paralyzed and unable to function. This sort of fear controls us. It also makes us particularly vulnerable to depression, panic attacks, and phobias.

What are we afraid of? What is it that we are actually afraid of if we suffer from this sort of paralyzing fear? We often think that we won't be able to cope, that whatever the situation is we will somehow fail. But the truth is that we are not wanting to re-experience that horrible feeling we unconsciously remember from childhood, that feeling of inadequacy brought about by being criticized, mocked, teased, and generally found wanting. We assume, without realizing it, that everyone in our adult life will treat us the same way that some in our childhood did.

Shyness Some of us are cripplingly shy. We are sure that other people look down on us and think we are less clever, attractive, or funny than they are. We are sure we will be rejected. This fear controls many of our decisions, from making friends and changing jobs, to joining in events that we might actually enjoy.

But the fear we live with is much, much greater than the fear we would experience if we would only take the risk. So, for example, go to the party you are scared of. You might get nervous and sweaty-palmed beforehand, feel butterflies in your stomach, convince yourself that everyone in the room is more socially adept than you, but go anyway. You might not enjoy the first party you go to, or even the second, but the fear *will* diminish. Each time you survive a room full of people you will feel better about yourself. You will realize they are not all cleverer or more socially adept than you. You will come to understand that you are worth as much as anyone else and may even discover that some of them are as frightened as you. You may decide that parties are not your thing, but you won't be scared of them anymore.

Phobias Many of us suffer from a phobia, which is an irrational fear that makes a sufferer do almost anything to avoid the subject of the phobia. These range from dental phobia and fear of flying to claustrophobia or the fear of open spaces. In bad cases people even consider life changes such as quitting their job, turning down promotion, or moving house to avoid their overriding fear. Cognitive Behavioural Therapy can be very successful in addressing phobias (see pages 108–9), as can Autogenic training, founded by German psychiatrist Dr Johannes Schultz in the 1920s. This therapy develops techniques to relax the body and calm the pulse, and can be directed at specific problems like phobias.

Rescue Remedy, one of the Bach flower remedies (see pages 64–5), helps to reduce the immediate anxiety of a phobia, or the feelings of panic we experience before we speak in public or sit an exam. There are even computer games, such as "Fear Fighter", which take an interactive approach to ridding us of our fears.

Confront it Whatever you are afraid of, the best way to get rid of the fear and stop it ruining your life is to confront it. This diminishes its potency and, although the situation that triggered the fear might always be something you would rather avoid, it will no longer have the power to stop you enjoying yourself.

Do it anyway
American psychologist Susan Jeffers says that one of the misconceptions we all labour under is that we will eventually stop experiencing fear. So often we avoid the challenges of new, different, and yes, scary, things in the hopes that we won't have to experience any more fear. But we have to accept that at times we will have a pounding heart and sweaty palms. If we carry on regardless to do what we fear most, the next time, hopefully, we won't be so afraid.

If we don't do things because we are afraid, then we will always remain scared of doing them.

Evidence
An American study in 1999, conducted by psychiatrists Richard Heimberg and Michael Liebowitz, took a group of people suffering from social phobia and compared those treated with drug therapy and those treated with Cognitive Behavioural Therapy. Both groups improved enormously (80% of people in each), but the CBT group only had a 17% relapse rate, while 50% of the people who had been on drug therapy relapsed.

Do you take life too seriously?

Do you know enough people who make you laugh?

Do you worry about being out of control?

Laughter therapy

"Cheer up, it might never happen" is a classic jibe and, irritating as the comment can be, it does make an important point. As adults we often tend to take life much too seriously. One study showed that four-year-olds laugh on average 500 times a day, but as adults our average is only 15. We forget how life-enhancing laughter is. When was the last time you laughed until you were out of control?

How it works
Laughter is said to increase cardiovascular flexibility because as we laugh both our blood pressure and pulse rise, then drop. Gulping in air as we laugh increases the oxygenation of our brain and body and also encourages the production of those all-important mood-enhancing endorphins.

Laughter workout
The American cognitive psychologist, Mariana Funes, suggests that we should find ourselves a laughter partner and then try laughing together for absolutely no reason for a full minute, or even longer, each one keeping the other one going. Don't laugh at anyone, or at anything, just learn to let go and laugh.

It is the common assumption that we laugh when we are happy. But if you think about it, we often laugh when we are nervous, shy, tense, or extremely sad too. It is a body process – like crying, yawning, or trembling – that allows us to release all sorts of emotions. We may laugh when we are with someone who shares our sense of humour, but this is just one of the many triggers.

Laughter connects
Laughing is one of the quickest ways to connect with others. If you work with a group of people who can all laugh together it makes your job much more pleasurable and the time goes a lot more quickly. If your family can laugh with each other, even in adversity, you are all much more likely to stay close.

Sharing embarrassments There is nothing more embarrassing than that moment when you realize that you have made a terrible mistake, seen something you shouldn't have seen, worn something or done something that you feel shames you. Most of us take these moments much too seriously. We see everyone laughing and want to die. But most of the people who are laughing are doing it automatically, due to the overwhelming sense of relief that it isn't happening to them. Most of them forget the incident almost as soon as it has happened. And each one of them will have faced exactly the same, or similar, embarrassments themselves. It can help to share these moments with others. Take turns to recount your most embarrassing moment, and laugh about it together.

Things that make you laugh We've all got laughter triggers; books, poems, films, sitcoms, or comedians that make us laugh. When you are feeling down, get out your favourite funny film or book and indulge yourself in some really deep laughing.

Laughing clubs and therapies A Bombay doctor instigated medicinal laughing clubs based on a yogic posture that is said to invoke laughter. Since the first club was set up in 1995, more than 100 have been established across India. The members meet in groups of about 50 and make one another laugh.

Patch Adams, an American doctor, almost ruined his career because of the opposition from his superiors in the 1980s about his belief that his cancer patients got better more quickly when he encouraged them to laugh. However, laughter therapy is now gaining ground in many American hospitals.

The funny side We all know that we feel better after we have had a laugh. Laughter releases tension, reduces anxiety, and also helps us when we are ill, so try to see the funny side of things more to increase the laughter quotient in your life.

Laughing with others

Much humour, unfortunately, is based on ridiculing others. Healing laughter is about laughing with someone, not at them. It is alright to tease someone close to you, who understands and is happy to share the joke. However, many of us have been the victims of unwarranted teasing, such as jokes about our appearance or intellectual capacity. Make sure your laughter is always based in kindness and not at the expense of others.

Evidence

A Californian study carried out in 1995, using 10 healthy male volunteers who were shown a humorous video, discovered that laughter lowered the levels of the stress-hormone cortisol in their blood, thereby protecting their immune systems.

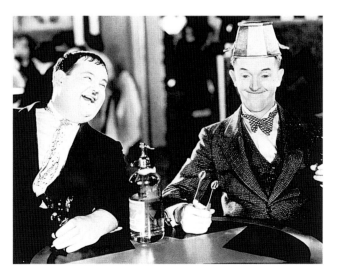

Laurel and Hardy ought to have been given medals for making us laugh so much, because the process of laughter has genuine benefits for our health.

Bibliography

Baggott, Andy, *The Encyclopedia of Energy Healing*, Godsfield Press (1999)

Ballentine, Rudolph, *Radical Healing*, Rider Books (1999)

Bloomfield, Harold, *Healing Anxiety with Herbs*, Thorsons (1998)

Bowlby, John, *Attachment and Loss*, Penguin (1981)

Bradford, Nikki (ed), *The Hamlyn Encyclopedia of Complementary Health*, Hamlyn (2000)

Briffa, John *BodyWise*, CIMA Books (2000)

Carter, Rita, *Mapping the Mind*, Seven Dials (1999)

Clarke, Jane, *Body Foods for Life*, Weidenfeld and Nicolson, Orion Publishing Group (1998)

The Dalai Lama, *Path to Tranquillity*, Rider (1998)

Davis, Patricia *Aromatherapy A–Z*, C W Daniel (1999)

Foundation for Inner Peace, *A Course of Miracles*, Viking 1996

Freke, Timothy, *Encyclopedia of Spirituality*, Godsfield Press (2000)

Funes, Mariana, *Laughing Matters*, Newleaf (2000)

Gilbert, Paul, *Overcoming Depression*, Robinson Publishing (1997)

Greenfield, Susan (ed), *Brain Power*, Element (2000)

Harvey, Clare and Cochrane, Amanda, *The Healing Spirit of Plants*, Godsfield (1999)

Holford, Patrick, *The Optimum Nutrition Bible*, Piatkus (1997)

Jeffers, Susan, *Feel the Fear and Do it Anyway*, Rider (1998)

Kewley, Michael, *Life Changing Magic*, Panna Dipa Books (1999)

LeDoux, Joseph, *The Emotional Brain*, Simon and Schuster (1996)

Ornish, Dean, *Love and Survival*, Vermilion (1998)

Rowe, Dorothy, *Depression*, Routledge (1996)

Sivananda Yoga Vedanta Centre, *Yoga Mind and Body*, Dorling Kindersley (1998)

Stuttaford, Thomas, *In Your Right Mind*, Faber and Faber (1999)

Styron, William, *Darkness Visible*, Picador (1991)

Swami Dayananda *Introduction to Vedanta*, Vision Books (1998)

Walsch, Neale Donald, *Conversations with God, Book I*, Hodder and Stoughton (1997)

Webb, Marcus and Maria, *Healing Touch*, Godsfield (1999)

Whiteaker, Stafford, *The Good Retreat Guide*, Rider (1998)

Wills, Judith, *The Food Bible*, Quadrille Publishing (1999)

Wolpert, Lewis, *Malignant Sadness*, Faber and Faber (1999)

Woodham, Annie and Peters, Dr David, *Encyclopedia of Complementary Health*, Dorling Kindersley (1997)

Useful addresses

Alcoholics Anonymous
Box 1, Stonebow House
Stonebow
York Y01 7NJ
Tel: 01904 644026
Helpline: 020 7833 0022
www.alcoholics-anonymous.org.uk

Association for Postnatal Illness
25 Jerdan Place
London SW6 1BE
Tel: 020 7386 0868
www.apni.org

Association of Reflexologists
27 Old Gloucester Street
London WC1N 3XX
Tel: 0990 673320
www.aor.org.uk

The Bach Centre
Mount Vernon
Bakers Lane
Sotwell
Wallingford OX10 0PZ
Tel: 01491 834678
www.bachcentre.com

British Acupuncture Council
63 Jeddo Road
London W12 9HQ
Tel: 020 8735 0400
www.acupuncture.org.uk

British Association of
    Psychotherapists
37 Mapesbury Road
London NW2 4HJ
Tel: 020 8452 9823
www.bap-psychotherapy.org

British Homeopathic Association
15 Clerkenwell Close
London EC1R 0AA
Tel: 020 7566 7800
trusthomeopathy.org

The British Massage Therapy
    Council
78 Meadow Street
Preston
Lancashire PR1 1TS
Tel: 01772 881063
www.jolanta.co.uk

British Medical Acupuncture Society
12 Marbury House
Higher Whitley
Warrington

Cheshire WA4 4QW
Tel: 01925 730727
www.medical-acupuncture.co.uk

Chinese Heritage Ltd
(Qigong)
Katana House
Shillingford Bridge
Shillingford
Oxfordshire OX10 8NA
Tel. 01865 858830

Cruse Bereavement Care
126 Sheen Road
Richmond
Surrey TW9 1UR
Tel: 020 8940 4818

Depression Alliance
35 Westminster Bridge Road
London SE1 7JB
England Tel: 020 7633 9929
Scotland Tel: 0131 467 3050
Wales Tel: 01222 521 774
www.depressionalliance.org.uk

Institute for Complementary
    Medicine
PO Box 194
London SE16 7QZ
Tel: 020 7237 5165
www.icmedicine.co.uk

The International Society of
    Professional Aromatherapists
82 Ashby Road
Hinckley
Leicestershire LE10 1SN
Tel: 01455 637987
www.the-ispa.org

Mental Health Foundation
20-21 Cornwall Terrace
London NW1 4QL
Tel: 020 7535 7400
www.mentalhealth.org.uk

MIND (National Association for
    Mental Health)
15-19 Broadway
London E15 4BQ
Mindinfoline: 0208 522 1728
Outside London: 0345 660 163
www.mind.org.uk

Narcotics Anonymous
PO Box 417
London SW10 0RP
Tel: 020 7351 6794

National Federation of Spiritual
    Healers (NFSH)
Old Manor Farm Studio
Church Street
Sunbury-on-Thames TW16 6RG
Tel: 01932 783164
www.nfsh.org.uk

The Nutricentre (Flower Remedies)
The Hale Clinic
Park Crescent
London W1N 3HE
Tel: 020 7436 5122

Royal London Homeopathic
    Hospital
Great Ormond Street
London WC1N 3HR
Tel: 020 7837 8833

SADA (Seasonal Affective Disorder
    Association)
PO Box 989
Steyning
West Sussex BN44 3HG
Tel: 01903 814942

The Samaritans
10 The Grove
Slough SL1 1QP
Tel: 01753 216500
Helpline: 0345 909090
www.samaritans.org.uk

School of Tai Chi Chuan
Centre for Healing
5 Tavistock Place
London WC1H 9SN
Tel: 020 8444 6445

Shiatsu Society
Eastlands Court
St Peter's Road, Rugby
Warwickshire CV21 3QP
Tel: 01788 555051
www.shiatsu.org

Sivananda Yoga Vedanta Centre
51 Felsham Road
London SW15 1AZ
Tel: 020 8780 0160
www.sivananda.org (general)
www.sivanandayoga.org (centre)

Society of Homoeopaths
4A Artizan Road
Northampton NN1 4HU
Tel: 01604 621400
www.homeopathy-soh.org

Index

Author's acknowledgments

I would like to offer sincere thanks to my family, the team at Mitchell Beazley, Claire Musters, Hagen Rampes, Judie Sandeman-Allen, and Richard Tyson, for their support on what has been a truly collaborative work.

Picture credits

7 Photonica/John Russell; 13 Getty One Stone; 19 bottom left Retna Pictures Ltd/Gavin Harrison; 29 bottom left Getty One Stone/Elie Bernage; 39 Retna Pictures Ltd/Howard Black; 47 Anthony Blake Photo Library/Tim Hill; 48 centre left Anthony Blake Photo Library/Maximillian; 49 bottom Anthony Blake Photo Library/ PFT Associates; 50 bottom right Getty One Stone/Ranald Mackechnie; 53 bottom left Octopus Publishing Group Ltd/Sandra Lane; 55 bottom left Octopus Publishing Group Ltd/Jeremy Hopley; 56 bottom Anthony Blake Photo Library/Maximilian; 61 bottom right Octopus Publishing Group Ltd/Edward Allwright; 62 bottom left Garden Picture Library/Howard Rice; 67 top left Image Bank/Anthony Edwards; 69 Getty One Stone/Dale Durfee; 71 bottom left Robert Harding Picture Library; 73 bottom right Getty One Stone/Bruce Ayres; 89 bottom left Getty One Stone/Mark Douet; 91 Getty One Stone/A & L Sinibaldi; 93 bottom right The Stock Market; 94-95 bottom Getty One Stone/Josh Mitchell; 99 bottom left Images Colour Library Limited; 109 top left Robert Harding Picture Library/Scott Barrow/Int'l Stock; 113 Getty One Stone/Ian O'Leary; 119 bottom left Octopus Publishing Group Ltd/Peter Myers; 129 Photonica/M. Grondahi; 130 bottom right Getty One Stone/Tom Stock; 135 top left Mark Azavedo Photo Library; 143 bottom left Images Colour Library Limited/National Geographic; 145 Getty One Stone/Jerome Tisne; 146 bottom right Retna Pictures Ltd/Luke White; 155 bottom right The Ronald Grant Archive